DISCLAIMER

This book is intended for your general knowledge only, to give valuable insight. It is not a substitute for a consultation and proper care by a medical doctor and should not be used as a tool to make a diagnosis. You must seek prompt medical attention for any health problems.

Printed in Australia

First Printing 2024

ISBN: 978-0-6453760-9-8

White Light Publishing

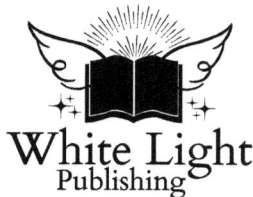

White Light
Publishing

www.whitelightuniversal.com.au

Heads Up

LEIGH RAY

Internationally Trained Expert Jaw Physiotherapist

All the information nobody wants to talk about for TMJ, Migraines, Headaches, Neck, Jaw, Ear & Sinus Pain

CONTENTS

Chapter 1   5
Jaw Pain & Dysfunction
Often mistook as ear pain, blocked feeling, fullness

Chapter 2   8
Migraines

Chapter 3   14
Headaches & Neck Pain

Chapter 4   21
Ear Pain & Tinnitus

Chapter 5   24
Kids - Clenching/Grinding Head/Tummy Pain

TREATMENT OPTIONS

Chapter 6   28
Diet, Detox, Elimination Trial - What food is making you sick?

Chapter 7   36
Vitamin Support

Chapter 8   39
Hormones

Chapter 9   46
Thyroid & Insulin Resistance
A big part of TMD, migraines and headaches

Chapter 10   49
Airways, Sinus & Saliva Glands

Chapter 11   53
Mouth Splints, Bruxism & Sleep Hygiene

Chapter 12   58
Pelvic Floor & Lower Back Pain

Chapter 13   61
Medications, Botox & Surgery

Chapter 14   64
Positive Parenting

Chapter 15   69
Quantum Physics or Brain Evolution

Biography   79
Leigh Ray - The Jaw Physio

Resources & References   81

Whole health options for people with jaw/TMJ, migraine, headache, neck, ear pain & noise. This guide is for the chronic pain people with these conditions, in simple terms, without the technical jargon, for simple lifestyle changes.

This book is intended for your general knowledge only, to give valuable insight. It is not a substitute for a consultation and proper care by a medical doctor and should not be used as a tool to make a diagnosis. You must seek prompt medical attention for any health problems.

The body's physical tissues (bones, muscle, nerves, cartilage, etc) will heal in 6 weeks to 3 months. Any pain passed this point is considered chronic pain and will take more than one option to allow the body to heal.

This is not an individualised plan. You will have to decide (with your family or doctors) what will work for you and for how long you need to apply these suggestions.

There are no guarantees in this book. It is up to your heart and mind to decide what is best for your situation and develop wisdom around your illness.

Hopefully these chapters allow you to put a lot of puzzle pieces together and give you a path to health.

In counselling they say, "whatever you hate doing the most (that is healthy), you probably need the most." So, whichever suggestion you find the hardest, they are probably the most important. But you don't have to do it in a correct order to get it right.

Start with small easy steps first to form healthy new habits and build up to the bigger changes as your brain gets used to a new paradigm shift.

Enjoy learning what works for you, what you're not ready for yet, but might do later. And put in the bin what doesn't work.

Please enjoy seeing the whole picture, or as much as I have been exposed to in my journey, as a therapist and "ex" chronic pain person. I'm sure I have missed parts. This book will be revised in time to reflect my learning.

When I comment on large trends (what works) in my clinic for my clients, it is based on clients I have treated in this area only, for the last 10 years, and general physio conditions and research I have been exposed to over the last 20 yrs. This means I only see a sub-section of these condition. I do not treat all presentations of these conditions, you will have to make your own decisions, I am NOT responsible for your healing, this is up to you. You need to make the choice to seek medical consultation.

If you are in crisis, this product is not to be used, please see your doctor or mental health specialist.

Healthdirect lines: https://www.healthdirect.gov.au/mental-health-where-to-get-help

CHAPTER 1

JAW PAIN & DYSFUNCTION
Often mistook as ear pain, blocked feeling, fullness

Jaw pain is very uncomfortable and can often be associated with ear pain, neck pain and face pain. Most clients experience: 'clicking' &/or 'locking' of their jaw, jaw pain and neck pain (associated with a 'worn out'/degenerative neck joints). Other symptoms can include; ear pain/pressure/dripping feeling/fluid feeling, tinnitus type sounds, headaches and grinding of teeth. Often anxiety, neck pain and headaches occur before the jaw pain.

Other common symptoms include:
- Pain on chewing, yawning or opening the mouth widely.
- Clicking noises on opening and closing the mouth.
- Difficulty or inability to open the mouth fully.
- Locking of the jaw.
- Thickness, fullness, fluid moving, blocked ears research shows that if you grinded your teeth as a kid, you will your whole life.
- Clinically TMD clients also report a long history of ear and or sinus infections.

Causes of Jaw Pain (Headaches & Migraines) are usually due to many conditions that have built up over the years.

Such as; Poor diet of unhealthy foods/processed, Sugar, caffeine, alcohol, drugs, breathing blockages (from chemical inflammation from disorders or poor diet or skeletal blockages), hormonal imbalance, auto immune conditions, malabsorbing guts/IBS/funny tummies, changing medications, poor sleep/insomnia, direct trauma to the area, posture, childhood templating (how you were brought up and the 10 generations behind your parents that cemented your belief system/ethics/morals), social interactions with partners/friends, etc.

Definition

The temporomandibular joint (TMJ) is the hinge joint that connects the lower jaw (mandible) to the temporal bone of the skull. Temporomandibular disorders (TMD) occur as a result of problems with the jaw bone/cartilage/disc, jaw joint, and surrounding facial muscles that control chewing and moving of the jaw.

Most often, I see it as the disc that is displaced/swollen (not sitting in the middle of the joint) or the disc is inflamed.

The overactive muscles are due to triggers in your life (i.e. poor diet, sugar, pollution, auto immune conditions, hormonal imbalance, mental health issues, feelings of isolation/loneliness, stress, too many work hours, funny tummies, poor sleep, negative social interactions, drugs, etc) and are secondary (or not the main reason) for creating the pain.

Treatment on this area should be gentle, not rough, and not overly painful. As most people with this condition have an over sensitive nervous system. If you are too strong with treatment, these symptoms are easy to exacerbate/make worse.

We have gentle exercises that allow your endurance muscles of the jaw to thicken/strengthen and help realign the jaw, creating an equal bite and ease of movement. See my online exercise course, or come into the clinic; DIY jawphysio Courses: *https://www.jawphysio.com.au/ diy-jawphysio-courses*

Clicking is very normal whilst you are strengthening these muscles and should eventually ease and stop. Clicking isn't considered a problem unless it hurts, or is a loud or big clunk.

Good Tips - Whilst in pain please avoid

- Yawning if it hurts to do so. (Yawning is good, just do it gently!) You usually yawn when tired, have tired/tight facial/jaw muscles and to lubricate the eyes. To help with yawning, just place the flat of your hands on either side of your jaws (like the painting, 'The Scream') and compress your joints, limiting how wide you open.

- Opening your mouth wide.
- Testing to see if it still clicks, locks.
- If your jaw locks up, try not to open your mouth up to that point.
- Avoid forcing your jaw to unlock - if your jaw locks on one side, often lying on one side will help it unlock - find out which side works for you.
- Sleeping on your stomach - (this sleeping position will mean constant therapy for your neck and jaw!).
- Working long hours.
- Talking a lot.
- Chewing gum (very bad for jaws in general), do not chew a pencil - this is very old fashioned advise that does NOT help.
- Going to the gym and using weights above shoulder height will aggravate your symptoms, so too will pec dec, lat pull down machines, push ups and stomach crunches. Just go for a walk, or do leg exercises, this area is sore, don't put more strain on it.

Exercise Tip

A little sneaky peak at Leigh's jaw and head pain exercise course available on her website *www.jawphysio.com.au* is the exercise called the 'Bullfrog.' If you have googled a lot, it is the exercise you do before the "N" exercise.

The Bullfrog switches off the masseter/cheek muscles and the swallow muscles that are overactive, and turns on the deep "Pilates" muscles either side of the joint, for combined (co contraction) to keep the jaw joint tracking in the centre, not deviating. Which reduces clicking, clunking and allows the jaw disc's to heal.

So just pop the tip of your tongue to the roof of your mouth, in the middle of the palate. Lips stay gently together, and open your jaw towards your throat (not forwards like a bulldog!!).

It is a small movement, your tongue may move away from the roof of your mouth.

Repeat 30 times, twice a day. And do just 2 every 30min, to stop you trying to touch your back teeth when you are concentrating.

CHAPTER 2

MIGRAINES

Migraines are still not fully understood, the guides are often too strict in classification, and migraines evolve/change over time.

Researchers used to think it was related to vascular structures (inflammation of blood vessels). Now they think it is related to an over sensitised central nervous system (the brain). Migraines are cyclical in nature and are very similar to Tension Type Headaches.

Over sensitisation, means too much information from the body, whether it be about the environment around the body, or the bodies internal process, all accumulate in one part of the brain, and it over flows (like an over flowing bucket), and the information/input flows into other parts of the brain and causes a migraine/head pain.

Both Migraine and Tension Type Headaches are inflammatory in nature, irritating the central nervous system (brain).

The classification is very large and confusing.

In the most basic form, migraines are usually one sided (of the head), easily aggravated with activity, aggravated by light/noise and very severe in pain intensity.

And can be with, or without aura.

This over sensitisation of the brain (in particular the cervico-trigmeinal nucleus) can be dampened down via the top 3 neck joints. The top 3 neck joints have nerves that feed forward into this area, the cervico-trigeminal nucleus. The Watson headache technique I am trained in, uses the top 3 neck joints, in gentle physiotherapy techniques, to dampen down the brain/central nervous system, (with no cracking of the neck).

30% of migraine sufferers will develop TMD/jaw pain!!!
Which triggers which????!!! A lot of dentists I speak
with, think it is the TMD/jaw pain triggering a lot of the
migraines. If you can heal or reduce the jaw pain, many
migraine sufferers say that their migraines are a lot less
intense and a lot less often. *(www.ichd-3.org)*

The medical profession uses triptan medication to control
migraines. It only works on 50% of suffers and will not
work at all if it is not taken early on. i.e. you must take the
medication at the first sign of a migraine, before nausea sets
in, otherwise it is useless. And yes, Botox is very effect for
this condition, however, you end up having to have it every
3-6 months for the rest of your life at $600-$1000 a sitting.

I think it is more important to find out why you are having
them, and quite frankly, migraine clients have way too
much going on in their lives, or brain thought patterns.
If you ask the psychologists 97% of the western world is
stuck in co-dependence. I think it is better to spend that
money on counselling, psychology and philosophy, finding
out why you can't stop that little voice inside of you putting
you down constantly ("critical parent voice"), or the "what
if questions" you constantly pose to yourself, and find out
who you are with no justification or need to apologise
for just being you. And this is what Leigh did, she spent
4 years working on co dependence and how to tame its
influence in her life, and funny enough all her chronic pain
has gone!!

I find most migraine sufferers have done a lot of research and
some know more about their condition than their doctor!

So to start with, migraines are complex and involve many
health factors.

A good start is by removing all chemicals from your house
(use eco-friendly products), **remove any mould** from your
house/work area/ especially bathrooms, **clean air con filters**
regularly, **see a nutritionist/naturopath** for your specific
body shape/metabolism requirements, diet changes, blood
pressure check-ups, sleep studies and airway restrictions/
sleep apnoea, and many many more considerations.

Most of Leigh's clients with TMD/Migraine/Tension type headaches have women's health conditions as well. Most of her clients have not had a blood test of their sex hormones (progesterone, estrogen, DHEA, and testosterone) to see if they are low.

Particularly low progesterone can lead to; headaches, migraines, TMD, bruxism, insomnia, body pain, fatigue, low mood, hot flushes, poor memory, poor brain attention span, and much more. As referenced by Dr Dan Pursers book, Progesterone, detailing how much more effective and safer bioidentical hormones are than the pill/HRT. Please see Dr Dan Purser website *(https://danpursermd.com)* for his research, information, safety, and prescription. You can email me for who I refer to in Australia (most have telehealth).

Resistance to medications can mean your brain needs a software update! And seeing a counsellor/psychologist can help work out how to change how your brain reads the information coming from your nerve endings in your body (in the simplest explanation). Quantum physics has proven spirituality/psycho-social factors are the same thing.

Science is no longer separate to the mind/universe connection. Basically, science has finally been able to measure the atom (99.9% energy, 0.01% mass), so your body is full of atoms, and thus is 99.9% energy. Therefore, what you think and feel (i.e. your personality or soul) is the determining factor to how you react to life, with pain, or with joy. Seeing a counsellor/spiritualist/pastor can help your brain change the way it interprets pain or a lack of it. You have the choice to change. Very exciting times. See more in the Quantum Physics and Brain chapter.

Some groundbreaking books on help with Migraines (aura and without aura): Progesterone, Dr Dan Purser

The secret language of your body, Inna Segal, will help give you a clue into your emotional ties around this pain. Part of the therapy from an injury is the emotional (not just physical and medication). It is up to you to seek the right spiritual therapy.

The body keeps the score, by Bessel van der Kolk (Psychotherapist).

Many people with migraines also suffer secondary headaches different to their migraine.

If the migraine pain pathway on your head is the same as your headache pathway, Leigh has a higher than higher success rate treating with hands on techniques.

If the migraine pathway on your head is different to the pain pathway of your headache, it is harder to treat.

If you are waking with migraines/headaches/neck, it's a big indication that its due to your night clenching/grinding (not a sign you need a new pillow!), usually due to sleep apnoea or a liver that needs detoxing (as hormones that are not effectively being broken down, get stored here), usually due to stress - cortical burn out!

Treatment:
The first part of the treatment; (For non aura migraines), in Leigh's clinic;
Is thought to dampen down the trigeminocervical complex via the upper neck joints, with firm pressure to firstly make sure the neck is in central alignment (i.e. no stiff joints or rotated neck joints, specifically C2 and C3).

We are finding it is most successful with people whose headaches become their migraines (i.e. as the headache gets worse, it becomes migraine pain, and the referral pattern is the same, without aura. This treatment works regardless of its triggers (stress, dehydration, menstrual, cluster etc).

The technique does not involve any 'cracking' of the neck joints, and we complete a thorough assessment to see if your symptoms are suitable for the technique. **Both the Physio and the client will know within x2-3 sessions whether it is working.** Usually I see the client x2 the first week and x2 the second week. If you have not had at least 50% reduction of symptoms we reassess and recommend a specialist to manage your case.

It is very importantly you do your home exercises, as our treatment is only half the treatment. The exercises help with your body awareness and a more central spinal position with everyday life.

Clients with migraines that are separate to their headaches (i.e. are on a different referral pathway on their head) are more difficult to treat. So too with menstrual related headaches/migraines and aura associated migraines.

These technique are safe on any age from 4 years old to 104 years old. We check that you have vital neck ligaments in tact before we work on your neck.

The second part of treatment; (Aura type migraines) Involves an extensive assessment and questioning of your medical background and biochemical pathways.

For example **restrictions in your airways** can increase your clenching and impact on your health.

Bad Guts! - Bad gut bacteria, gut anaemia, lots of different gut conditions can impact on your health, including increasing your clenching.

In Leigh's clinic, a portion of migraine women have immediately got rid of their migraines from reducing or stopping gluten intake. More on this in the Diet Chapter.

Hormonal Imbalances - For women, changes in hormone levels; (from stress, sugar, pollutants; diesel/plastics), to normal teenage hood, menopause, pregnancy, Endo, Polycystic ovary syndrome, menopause, will see an increase in your normal clench reflex day and or night.

Usually progesterone is the first hormone used to treat the imbalance. You can find out by having a simple blood test for; progesterone, oestrogen, DHEA, testosterone. Dr Dan Purser and in Leighs clinic, we are finding that bio identical progesterone is the best to reduce; all over body pain/fibromyalgia, migraine, TMD, hot flushes, low mood, insomnia and it is safe. Dr Dan Purser book - Progesterone, is a great resource for the bio identical progesterone safety and prescription (more in the hormone chapter).

For men, low testosterone can lead to floppy airways and thus restricted airways. Get your GP to check with a simple blood test. If you are overweight, your GP will not look at a hormone screening test, you must get your weight down.

Therefore, we assess your health and prioritise which specialist you should see to address each medical condition that could be contributing to your overall over activity of night and day clenching and over stimulation of the trigeminal nerve.

CHAPTER 3

HEADACHES & NECK PAIN

Headaches

You can experience just headaches, or with migraines, or from neck pain, or as your jaw pain gets worse.

The myofascial headache (tension headache) are a lot more prevalent than previously thought and shown in the evidence. Especially when associated with TMJ disorders, bruxism and cervicogenic headaches.

People with headaches do not often present with one simple musculoskeletal source. It is usually a more complex combination of factors, and a combination of therapies can be needed to relieve the symptoms.

People with headaches, orofacial pain and bruxism provide a complex 'story' as there are so many structures which can be responsible for their symptoms/pain.

Most headache sufferers know more than their therapists and there are over 300 classifications, see *www.ichd-3.org* for all the definitions.

Many headache people suffer different types of headaches, most likely 2 different types.

Any chronic sufferers of headaches can also develop secondary anxiety or depressive features compounding (making worse) the clients symptoms/presentation.

Neck related Headaches;

C0-1 Pattern - Band around head, above eyebrows, top of crown and up and over ears from base of skull (occiput), and often a feeling of ear blockage.

C1-2 Pattern - Through eyebrows, tear duct areas, then moves diagonally up to crown down to neck/back of skull. Band over top of head (feels like a hot on the head). Can be one sided or both.

C2-3 Pattern (most common) - Upper traps/neck and up and overhead to behind eyes, sinus areas of face, significant nausea and vomiting as well. Can be one sided or both **combination of 2 of the above can occur as well.**

Most of Leigh's clients with TMD/Migraine/Tension type headaches have women's health conditions as well. Most of these clients have not had a blood test of their sex hormones (progesterone, oestrogen, DHEA, and testosterone) to see if they are low.

Particularly low progesterone in women can lead to; headaches, migraines, TMD, bruxism, insomnia, body pain, fatigue, low mood, hot flushes, poor memory, poor brain attention span, and much more. (You don't have to have all of the symptoms). Low progesterone or high estrogen leads to high inflammation in the body and thus increased clenching and joint inflammation. See Dr Dan Purser book on Progesterone, the natural hormone, details on its safety and prescription, and the chapter on hormones in this guide.

Jaw Headaches
Will present as temple pain radiating up from the jaws and can radiate down into the neck. Or just in the temples. Also, you can get headaches from upper neck to up over their ears, or just over their ears.

According to Gwen Jull's work (Physiotherapist with PhDs on neuromuscular dysfunction in the neck, headache and migraines), her latest research shows that 60-80% of migraine sufferers have;

1) Cervical spine segmental dysfunction (neck issues) - cervical muscle dysfunction arising from muscular skeletal disorder (and neck muscle issues)

2) TCN (trigeminal cervical nucleus) sensitisation, (sensitised nervous system).

Treatment for Part 1
Clients with head/jaw pain will load through their joint surfaces first before muscle's (as all muscle reactions are delayed). Thus, clients often spend a lot of time

talking about their sore shoulders and knots, and about their sore shoulders associated with headaches and migraines. Shoulder (upper trapezius muscle) pain is related to compression through the top neck joints = C0-1 segments. They are situated just behind the jaws and often become inflamed when the jaw is inflamed. When palpated (touched by a therapist), they most often do not feel tight or knotty, they are long and weak from the pain inhibiting (switching them off) and making them weaker. With pain, clients often slump and wiggle all day long trying to get away from the pain. It is vital to learn how to strengthen lower trapezius (and lower back muscles for long-term sitting at work), and hold the spine up with good posture and stop overloading the neck. And thus, better posture and no fidgeting!!!! These muscles work at 20% all day long. So, practicing the posture exercises is to be done every 30 min for only 10-30 seconds. Often client's shoulders are taped into position to help with the exercise and find an immediate reduction in pain. Ask your therapist. Or see our exercise course at *https://www.jawphysio.com.au/diy-jawphysio-courses*

Treatment for Part 2
I can't rave enough about the Dean Watson Headache regimen. It has literally changed thousands of client's pain. You can look up therapists that do this technique on his website. *https://watsonheadache.com/*

If you have jaw involvement, you will have to find a jaw physio/therapist as well.

Most clients who suffer TMD/jaw pain will have radiating pain into their temples, causing a headache. Once the jaw joint inflammation (disc or synovitis) is treated, the headache will go away. Note - acupuncturing the temporalis muscle whilst the jaw joint is inflamed will give the client a massive headache. A sore temporalis on palpation is part of the diagnostic testing of TMD/temporomandibular disorder (under international standards the test is called Axis 1), it is not the structure responsible for the client's pain. Make sure you see someone who treats this area all the time, as people just working on your muscles will miss a lot of the structures responsible for your pain.

Night Clenching and Grinding Headaches
Headaches that come on immediately with waking up in the morning are due to restricted airways at night, either from airway collapse or inflammation of the body and airways.

Everyone on the planet clenches, however different medical conditions can increase this clench reflex, which causes the jaw pain and headaches. If your headaches are only on waking, it is from excessive clenching at night.

Traditionally the treatment has been to prescribe low dose anti-depressants to treat the nerve pain, a night splint (like a mouth guard), +/- Botox for quick pain relief (but this doesn't treat the cause of the increase clenching). The evidence shows that jaw pain/TMD is cyclical and will return in 6 months to 2 years with this treatment.

Or you can look at your whole life and create healthy living.

Change your diet to suit your age/lifestyle (stop the sugar, processed foods, and increase vegetables (x4-6 cups a day), increase fruits, less caffeine, less alcohol, no drugs, exercise kindly and often (remember cardio for over 40 yr olds does NOT get rid of fat), hobbies, life-work balance, meditate, have gratitude (diary or dinner table discussion), get blood tests and see where your biochemistry is low (take supplements), have counselling/psychology/philosophical study.

And you might need a splint whilst you spend 6 months doing this, until you are healthy enough to support your own airway and have stopped making your body an inflammatory skin sac! Yes, negative thoughts do release inflammation and reduce serotonin production (happy vibe chemical in your body).

Sleep studies can be helpful. But remember the CPAP machines only work for 30-40% of the population. You can trial different masks and change the settings on the machine regularly with your sleep Doctor to make sure you are optimising the machine. The above (healthy living) is also vital, and a life saver for the 60% that can't use the CPAP machines. *https://headachejournal.onlinelibrary.wiley.com/ doi/10.1111/head.13816?fbclid=IwAR1n1LwF8_FcbiHqZZVPh1Os bTWrgzMPxSeXpC5DtFW0RMb-MSnntm7TZ_0*

Clinically we are noticing triggers for increased clenching at night (bruxism): Gastrointestinal problems (leaky gut, IBS, anaemia etc), respiratory blockages (deviated septum, rhinitis, polyps etc), change in hormones (teenage years, menopause, pregnancy etc), changes in medication, alcohol usage, and more.

We are also noticing clinically, triggers which increase your day clenching;

Increased use of computer screen use, poor posture, concentrating, stress.

Lack of Sleep and Headaches:
It is important to note that headaches may also be associated with respiratory sleep disorders such as limitation of airflow (upper resistance syndrome, UARS), or cessation of breathing (sleep apnoea) (Gold et al 2003).

We now know that a lack of sleep will increase your pain levels and thus you suffer from more headaches. Which starts first, less sleep due to pain of headaches, or the other way round. Both are true and impact on your pain and headaches. Reference; *(www.tmj.org/hope-in-research/ landmark-studies/oppera-study)*.

OTHER REASONS

Diet
New research into diet and repeated use of anti-biotics as a child are showing alteration in gut biomes, which can cause an over activity of nitrate producing bacteria which in turn produce nitric oxide, which causes Vaso dilation of blood vessels and can create head pain.

Gluten intolerance (never mind allergies and coeliac) are great at giving headaches and migraines. Many of my clients, by coming off gluten for 3 months have changed their lives for the better. Why are we now intolerant to gluten? We have genetically modified our wheat so that we can harvest it when it gets to 1m high. Whereas natural wheat, we used to have to wait until it was 2 m high. Natural wheat is still grown in Italy and Egypt, that's why when you travel overseas you don't get the same bloated tummy, weight gain and funny tummies, as its not genetically modified.

Auto immune disorders often come with headaches (as they are inflammatory conditions, reduce you inflammation in your body with diet changes, counselling to reduce negative self-talk, no alcohol/coffee, reduce work hours, gentle exercise, sleep routine, etc), e.g. Lupus, Endometriosis, Ehrlos Danlos, Autism, etc.

Hormonal Imbalances - For Women, Endo, Polycystic ovary syndrome, menopause, etc.

Usually, progesterone is the first hormone used to treat the imbalance. You can find out by having a simple blood test for - progesterone, oestrogen, DHEA, testosterone. I am seeing that my clients respond better to natural grade/bio identical progesterone to reduce; all over body pain/fibromyalgia, migraine, TMD, hot flushes, low mood, insomnia and it is safe.

Dr Dan Pursers website and books talk about their safety and prescription, Dan Purser MD, see more in my hormone chapter.

Hormonal Imbalances - Research in men with sleep apnoea found that a mild drop in testosterone (not enough to cause libido drop) can lead to floppy airways and thus restricted airways. In females our equivalent is Progesterone.

Gut Disorders - Anaemia, leaky gut, IBS.

Sinus Headaches (very rare) - More due to C1/2 neck pain referral pain, allergies, drinking milk.

A good remedy for sinus, taught to me by a naturopath is the combination of garlic/horseradish/vit C in one tablet at three times the dosage for 2 weeks, rest for 2 weeks and repeat if needed.

Most of the ENTs in Perth refer to me and they all recommend to their clients to cut out cow's milk, with sinus issues. Remember soy milk is an estrogen-based product, so it is not good if you are a jaw pain person, as most women are low progesterone, making estrogen more dominant (which is your high inflammation hormone). You want to bias your foods on progesterone foods, and not increase estrogen. Estrogen causes inflammation, gives you sugar cravings and reduces the good work of progesterone. See the hormone chapter for more info.

CHAPTER 4

EAR PAIN & TINNITUS

Why does my ear hurt? I can hear noises, even similar to tinnitus? Or I can hear/feel dripping/fluid and there is nothing coming out, or fluid is coming out.

WARNING: If you have fluid coming out of your ear, please see a doctor immediately. Most of the time it is fine, but you can aid it with grommets and or better diet. You just need to make sure it's not an infection or the rare case of cerebral spinal fluid, or any other condition.

If the GP has repeatedly syringed your ear and you can still feel/hear fluid, and grommets have not worked, you will need to see a Jaw Physio.

The rear portion of the jaw joint is separated from the front wall of the external ear canal by a thin plate of bone. Both the ear and the jaw receive nerves from the same branch (trigeminal nerve, which becomes the auriculotemporal nerve). So inflammation on this nerve can refer to the jaw and the ear, or both at the same time.

An inflamed jaw joint or displaced jaw joint (due to disc injury/degeneration) can be displaced backwards into the ear canal (Selesnick et al 1995) In some people there may be an absence of this thin plate of bone, thus more noise is heard in the ear from the vibration or noises of the jaw joint.

Or, it can be due to pain from the throat (tonsils, larynx, pharynx), in this case the ear pain occurs after swallowing,

Or, neck muscles closely inserting near the ear, most commonly the sternocliedomastoid muscle.

Often described by clients that their hearing has a feeling 'fullness' or 'pressure.' (Simons et al 1990).

Tinnitus - Has no identifiable cause. Sometimes it can be related to the above or even, the internal ligaments of the ear and jaw.

The oto-mandibular ligaments are the discomalleolar ligament (DML), which arises from the malleus (one of the ossicles of the middle ear) and runs to the medial retrodiscal tissue of the TMJ, and the anterior malleolar ligament (AML), which arises from the malleus and connects with the lingula of the mandible via the sphenomandibular ligament. The oto-mandibular ligaments may be implicated in tinnitus associated with TMD.

A positive correlation has been found between tinnitus and ipsilateral (same side) TMJ disorder. It has been proposed that a TMJ disorder may stretch the DML and AML ligaments, thereby affecting middle ear structure equilibrium "It thus seems that otic symptoms (tinnitus, otalgia (ear pain), dizziness and hypoacusis) corresponding to altered ossicular spatial relationships (such as conductive middle ear pathologies) can also be produced from masticatory system pathologies." From *https://www.physio-pedia.com/TMJ_Anatomy*

Most commonly caused by age, or side effects to medication. Thus, as we age, more medications are prescribed, so more chance of tinnitus developing. Try to use good diet and exercise to heal the body rather than medications. Good natural hormones (not medical HRT) is very effective at allowing calcium to uptake into bones, so less arthritis/inflammation, and reduces cardiac events, rather than using statins etc (See Dr Dan Purser, Menopause book).

It is thought that chronic tinnitus is more related to how the brain interprets feedback from the rest of the body - i.e. our nervous system.

We know people who have busy minds, i.e. with traces of anxiety, worry, depression etc develop tinnitus.

Here is the article: *http://media.campaigner.com/ media/75/755191/2019%20Fall%20Journal%20Articles/ Autonomic%20and%20Psuchologic%20Risk%20factor%20 for%20Deve.pdf*

Usually, it is a loud ringing in the ears and may keep you awake at night. It may interfere with your ability to hear. It does reduce as your body finds a way to cope and starts to only be noticeable if you stop and listen for it or are tired/fatigued or distressed. It is likely to fade with time.

Going to bed at night with gentle/soft music (classical is the best type, or nature sounds) can help you adapt, and get to sleep.

Playing white noise for a few months can help reset the nervous system to lower the tinnitus noise.

Apple app = Noizes has nature sounds.

In counselling they say, 'Who's not listening to you'?

Or

"What are you not listening to that your body is trying to tell you"?

Most tinnitus people have a profound reaction to those 2 statements. Write it down, do some journalling, and create healthy loving boundaries to support self-care. What is simple self-care, 'do I need water/food/toilet/rest' rather than finishing an endless list of jobs.

So, a mixture of good, work life balance, boundaries spoken with loving kindness for self-first. Better diet, less alcohol/drugs, more joy activities and brain evolution (counselling, spirituality, self-development books, meditation etc).

I like the Buddhist philosophical saying, "nothing stays the same", something else will come up that will stop the tinnitus from being a priority!

CHAPTER 5

KIDS
Clenching/Grinding, Head/Tummy Pain

Dummies, pacifier, thumbs in your mouth all decrease your child's airways and increase grinding, clenching and future health problems.
Orthodontists have researched the use of the above and know that they all increase the palate arch as it grows. This decreases the amount of air the child breaths in and creates grinding, clenching, snoring, noisy breathing.

Source: *www.aamsinfo.org* Academy Of Applied Myofunctional Sciences.

Better palate formation in children with a simple exercise;
Throat muscle exercises - Pharyngeal dilator exercises, which is also great for low vagus tone, used by Buddhist monks is an ancient chant over 2600 years ago! Is;

Saying the following syllables very quickly, over and over again can help.

OM - AH - HUM
Start with 1 min continuously and build up to 10 - 15min x2/day - do it in the car on the way to school!

New Emerging Research;

OSD - Obstructive Sleep Disorder; otherwise known as restrictive airways, is one of the biggest contributors for excessive grinding and clenching at night.

So a referral to a sleep clinic and or ENT would be the first step. You will need a referral from your GP.

Peak development of the palate (roof of your mouth) is birth to 6yrs of age.

In this time breastfeeding and textured food is important in palate and pharyngeal (throat) development.

Then again at puberty.

Malocclusion in children (occlusion = the ability to meet the teeth, especially with eating) with no breastfeeding seems to be more prevalent.

Best to breastfeed for up to 6mth – to 12mths to protect against malocclusion.

Children learn nasal breathing and lip seal with breastfeeding.

If dummies/pacifiers are introduced, it negates the good effects of breast feeding.

Persistent nasal obstruction is usually due to high arch palate in children. May need oral facial surgery as well as a palate expansion device. Using palate expanders can increase the airflow up to 4 times to nasal.

Moderate to mild restricted airways can lead to orthodontists or specialist dentists for assessment of palate expanders. Indications for this are high shaped palates, noisy breathing, connective tissue/auto immune conditions which contribute to floppy airways.

Results of delayed speech with tongue tie and or use of dummy.

Jaws stop growing in females aged 14 - 16 years, in males 16 - 20 years, therefore they can be considered for surgical repair. And natural hormone therapy can commence to support airways (see Dr Dan Pursers book on Progesterone).

Cows Milk
This is a tough subject. The science says there is no link with milk and an increase in mucus production.

Most of the children I see have seen a Perth ENT and most of them will recommend coming off dairy for recurrent ear infections, jaw pain and increased clenching and grinding at night and skin rashes.

As too will most of these client's naturopath's, nutritionists, and nurse practitioners.

Here is some great information:

- Cow's milk protein is one of the most common causes of food allergy in children.
- Cow's milk protein (dairy) allergy is not the same as having lactose intolerance.
- Most children outgrow cow's milk protein allergy between 3-5 years of age.
- Allergy symptoms can appear on the skin, in the gut and/or respiratory system.
- Removing all dairy products, including cow's milk, from their diet may help with initial management of the food allergy and should be done in consultation with their healthcare professional.
- Finding appropriate substitutions for cow's milk and dairy products is important to help your child to meet their energy and nutritional needs.
- Reference: Milk - Allergy & Anaphylaxis Australia *(allergyfacts.org.au)*

Tongue Tie

Another condition that can create palate formation problems and thus can reduce the amount of air the child receives. It will also disrupt how a child learns to lip seal and suck and co-ordinate breathing with eating and drinking. It is important to get this assessed. And even more importantly to get it re accessed a few years after any operations, as they are often a conservative procedure, and your child might need another procedure. I find the dentists with extra training in sleep medicine very good and can do the procedure in the dentist chair with a laser.

Source: *www.aamsinfo.org* Academy Of Applied Myofunctional Sciences.

White Food

Fussy eaters through to Autistic children are really difficult for parents to handle. I often see children with ear pain, ear bleeding, jaw pain, grinding and they are only able to tolerate bland food. Often no vegetables and not much meat. Not only will this cause ear and jaw problems, but it will also lead to serious health conditions later on in life. Positive parenting courses - the autism WA website has great courses, seeing a dietician/nutritionist/paediatrician can be very helpful. Some helpful sites; Lit Therapy, Perth Kids hub, Western kids. Also getting your children to grow their own vegetables, to form a connection with planet and plant. Feel the effort and bond with their 'baby trees/food' to desensitise. And create an exciting adventure, to help pick the vegetables for the dinner plate that night. Also allows for fantastic gut biome exploration with being in the dirt... research shows better immunity and better cognition development with exploring the outside environment. Sources; *www.autism.org.au, perthkidshub.com.au, www.littherapy.com.au*

CHAPTER 6

DETOX, DIET, ELIMINATION TRIAL
What food is making you sick?

Detox
So many pollutants lead to headaches, migraine, sinus issues, colds, flu's, immunity problems etc.

Mould - Huge contributor to chronic pain, fatigue, headaches, lung conditions etc. Remember bleach products that say they are mould cleaners, only actually bleach the spores. Bleach does not kill all spores. And can be quite toxic to humans and animals/pets. If you can't afford to have it professionally cleaned. It's simple to just use white vinegar.

Further reading on how to clean mould from your house, see *https://www.betterhealth.vic.gov.au/health/conditionsandtreatments/mould-removal-at-home*

Remember to wear protective clothing and a mask. Do not allow vulnerable people in the area (no kids, pregnant women, immune compromised people).

Aircon filters, on split systems inside should be washed every 3 months, outside compressors of split systems need to be free from anything (garden stuff etc) and usually tolerate a good hose down 3 monthly (check your warranty/instruction manual).

Use natural cleaning products instead of chemicals.
You should never have to use bleach, it is toxic to humans, and our oceans/water ways and gardens. Simple cleaning hacks (from the bathroom to the drains in your house, don't forget to regularly clean your tooth brush, it doesn't get clean, cleaning your teeth!!!): *www.webmd.com/a-to-z-guides/ss/slideshow-guide-to-natural-cleaning, www.goodhousecleaning.com*

There are lots of sites on google and you can also add some essential oils, my favourite is immune boost from revive oils.

Products to avoid:

- **Formaldehyde** - This is a preservative that is often seen in lotions, cosmetics, and baby wipes. It's a known carcinogen and can cause skin and respiratory irritations.

- **Phthalates** - These are a group of chemicals found in personal care products and many plastics and vinyls. They can affect your endocrine system, reproductive health, and even potentially cause cancer.

- **VOCs** - Volatile organic compounds (VOCs) are gases that are emitted into the air. They're found in some building materials, home and personal products, gasoline, and even things like glue and permanent markers. Breathing VOCs can cause eye, nose and throat irritation as well as difficulty breathing and nausea, even damage to the central nervous system and other organs. Some VOCs can even cause cancer.

- **Sodium Lauryl Sulfate (SLS) and Sodium Laureth Sulfate (SLES)** - These are surfactants commonly used as an emulsifying cleaning agent in household cleaning products (laundry detergents, spray cleaners, and dishwasher detergents). In other words they keep things mixed up and help them create lather. Oftentimes they are synthetically derived and have the potential to cause skin irritation.

- **Ethanolamines (MEA, DEA, and TEA)** - These are found in many household and personal care products and have been linked to organ system toxicity, bioaccumulation, and even cancer.

- **Triclosan** - This is found in many antibacterial soaps, hand sanitizers, and detergents as well as some toothpastes, deodorants, cosmetics, plastics, and more. It can affect the thyroid and endocrine system and was recently banned by the FDA to be used in "antiseptic washes" but can still be found in some other products like toothpaste, cosmetics, and even clothing, kitchenware, furniture, and toys.

- **Fragrance** - The word "fragrance" can appear on a label and contain an enormous list of ingredients that a company is not required to disclose, as it is considered a 'trade secret.' That means a product could contain some awful ingredients and the consumer wouldn't even know! These chemicals could be linked to cancer, reproductive and developmental toxicity, allergies and sensitivities. Why take the risk?

Reduce your time in polluted environments.
Big pollutants are **Highways/freeways: Bitumen, Diesel, and petrol fumes create disease and are toxic up to 100-500m either side of a main highway.**

Research shows that the most toxic place to exercise is beside a freeway. Please do not use the cycle pathways to exercise beside freeways and highways. Try not to live close to a highway. Plant lots of trees on your verge/garden if you do, google which trees are super absorbers of pollution like silver birch trees.

Headaches, nausea, are very common when driving in high density traffic and highways.

https://www.lung.org/clean-air/outdoors/who-is-at-risk/highways

https://www.ncbi.nlm.nih.gov/pmc/articles/PMC1971259/

Reduce your time driving to work on freeways (use public transport, or go the long way off main roads, work from home!), go earlier and exercise before work, make breakfast at home and take to a park near work. Add your meditation in the park after breakfast.

Turn off your car if you are stationary (not at the lights!!), how many of us leave the car running whilst looking up an address on our phones. It pollutes us and the gardens around us. If you're like me, you try to grow as much of your own food as possible. And we don't want these fumes travelling into our homes, and offices.

Water

A lot of our water is full of heavy metals, too much chlorine, and many other things not healthy for us. Some of the pipes water flows through are copper and that erodes the zinc in our bodies (zinc is essential for hormone and immunity support).

So get a really good water filter. You pay for quality. I just put a whole system on my mains tape outside my house. Now all my taps have filtered water and what a change to my health. I felt very dizzy the first week (detox), and I've noticed I have a feeling of getting enough water into my body, whereas previously I didn't.

When they tested my water, the chlorine alone was 8 time higher than recommended levels. Chlorine also increases with increased temperature, so all that extra absorption in the shower over your whole body can lead to symptoms of headache, skin irritation, hair brittleness etc...

Organic vegetables, local farmers market, farmer direct meat n Veg (order online & home delivery for ease)

I think this is self-evident these days, with all the genetic changes in food showing poor gut absorption and all the build-up of 'sprays'/toxins in the environment. More nutrient rich, taste better, often cheaper.

My local farmer, is $40 for a big box of 'seasonal' veggies, *http://www.glavocichproduce.com.au*

And I order my meat from *www.ourcow.com.au* or *www.dirtycleanfood.com.au*

Great webinar by a favourite naturopath of mine on what chemicals disrupt our biological processes, especially hormones *https://www.youtube.com/watch?v=W3OAS65Yf_g*

Diet

This information I have sourced from naturopaths, nutritionists, dieticians I refer to and work with. It is all basic information to get you started whilst you wait to get into one of them for a more detailed and individualised plan.

There is no one plan fits all. But you can start the clean-up phase before you go and build a more educated food plan based on your deficiencies (ideal; CMA intracellular vitamin testing, Dan Purser MD home page for details), age, gender (i.e. hormones), and conditions.

Add Antioxidants to your food, as we live in a very polluted environment.
Google is great with which foods. *www.stjohns.health/documents/content/top-20-foods-high-in-antioxidants.pdf*

Eat foods in season! Basic but true. There is a lot of science supporting food that is nutrient rich when in season, in their own habitat, amongst a mixture of plants/balanced ecosystem, as opposed to being grown in greenhouses as a singular mass. Order from your local farmer. I order a big box of veggies for $40 from a farmer 5min away from me in suburbia. So much better than going to the shops.

Add micro greens - for 'Detox' or just boost your immunity

Add micro greens; Radish, arugula, broccoli, sunflower, kale, beet, peas, spinach, and mustard microgreens are highly nutritious, containing essential vitamins A, B, C, E, K, minerals calcium, iron, magnesium, and potassium, sulforaphane, and antioxidants such as anthocyanins and quercetin, beta-carotene and lutein. Reference: *www.microgreensworld.com*

The following is not a supplement diet, it is a trial to see what products are making you sick, or how much of each food product can you tolerate before you give yourself symptoms.

For me, I can only eat pasta x1-2/week, more than that and I get bloating and brain fog. But I had to clean up my system for 3 months before I could make a scientific measurement of each food product.

Reduce / STOP Sugar!!!! For 3 months

We all know this, but its SOOO hard. But worth it. I have had many naturopaths, and nutritionists start me and my clients on this advice, and I got my life back (no bloating, no funny tummies, brain fog went, memory came back, stinky farts stopped!!! The list goes on).

Stop sugar for 3 months. No processed foods, no complex sugars (no pasta, no rice, no bread), no tomato sauce/BBQ sauce etc. Put it all in the bin now. Don't wait to use it up, as you will just buy more!

What do you eat?, Meat and veggies at nearly double the serving you usually have if you use a lot of pasta and rice in your main meals. Slow cookers are great and so healthy.

My favourite is lamb shank, broccolini, pumpkin, rosemary (rosemary really aids gut absorption).

> Note: If you are estrogen dominant, it is a researched fact you will not be able to stop craving sugar. Make sure your hormones are checked and corrected with bio identical hormones, *www.danpursermd.com* tells you why on his website and books. Reference: Understanding Estrogen Dominance, Lawley Hormone Solutions booklet, *www.lawleypharm.com.au*

No Gluten - no bread, no pasta. For 3 months

At the end of 3 months, slowly re introduce one food at a time and you will find your limit. Most of us are intolerant to pasta, as it has been genetically modified to be harvested at a quicker rate. Research shows our tummies just can't absorb it as well as the original wheat, and thus we don't feel well, brain fog, bloating, headaches etc. I know I can only have pasta x1-2/week, without symptoms. Obviously coeliac (intolerant to any gluten), needs specific testing, see *www.coeliac.org.au*

No Dairy - No milk, no cheese. For 3 months.
At the end of 3 months, slowly re introduce one food at a time and you will find your limit. Most of us have a limit to the amount we can tolerate. Find what is yours. Most ENT's will recommend no cow's milk (adults and kids) if you have sinus and ear issues.

You can stop all 3 at the same time. **Warning**, you will not feel well for the first 2 weeks, this is normal as you remove bad bacteria from your body, and mucosal lining blockages. It can come out as diarrhoea, postnasal drip (out of nose and ears), headaches, nausea, vomiting. Go with one elimination if you feel too unwell. Which is a good thing, because you have just found out what is making you feel so unwell.

Vegetables - 6 cups a day!
Nutritionists and Dieticians will recommend 6 cups of vegetables a day for healthy living. That means you need to up your intake at every meal and try and add them with breakfast.

Breakfast - Veggies in omelettes, smoothies, Mediterranean type breakfast - veggie sticks (carrot, cucumber, tomatoes etc).
Lunch - Salads, vegetable sticks with dips
Dinner - Double the amount of vegetables you usually cook.

I also like to do a month or 2 of low oxalate vegetables (google it), this will lower your sulphur intake and can help reduce systemic inflammation. Most imbalances come from poor knowledge of dosage amounts for types of foods. That's why we need to see an expert to tell you how much of each type of food you can eat for your genetics, conditions, energy output etc.

The Royal Prince Alfred Hospital Diagnostic Elimination Diet
For food intolerances. My clients who have failed everything and still have migraines and headaches have found this to be life changing. Warning it does really limit what you eat.
Reference: The RPAH Elimination Diet | The Failsafe Diet

(*https://www.failsafediet.com/lander*),
And Contact Us - The Gut Foundation
(*https://gutfoundation.com.au/contact-us/*)

Coffee - Only one a day between 11am and 3pm
Coffee later than 3pm, really effects sleep and significantly increases your clenching at night. Before 11am and you are using it to poo, creating a lazy bowel. You should naturally poo in the morning to clear your system for the day. Obviously, water first thing in the morning at least one glass of water after waking is vital to lubricate/hydrate your system, especially if you are a mouth breather.

Reference: OPPERA Study - *www.tmj.org/hope-in-research/landmark-studies/oppera-study*

Alcohol - Really increases your clench reflex
Try to just have it Friday to Sunday, and just one glass at a time. AAA and Alanon are great support services for people dealing with alcohol and are finding the sugar addiction too much for a start. Addiction is a big part of the Australian culture, most TV adds are based on having alcohol to be social or to relieve stress.

Most people are unaware that addiction is classed as the inability to stop, once you start the product; alcohol/sugar/chocolate/coffee/drugs etc Addiction habits that wont stop are strongly linked to child development from the age of 0 - 18 months of age, according to psychological paradigms. Seek understanding first before you judge yourself or others. Most clients I treat change when their kids become teenagers and they are being triggered back to their own teenage selves, and are seeing destructive communication patterns.

Reference:
OPPERA Study - *www.tmj.org/hope-in-research/landmark-studies/oppera-study*

Alcoholics Anonymous - Alcoholics Anonymous *(aa.org.au)*

Home - Al-Anon Family Groups (Australia) Pty Ltd
(*https://al-anon.org.au*)

CHAPTER 7

VITAMIN SUPPORT

Warning
A lot of the vitamin companies are now owned by big pharma. Many companies are reducing potency or number of tablets and increasing prices. Make sure you check the dosage on the back of your vitamin bottles, many of them are reduced potency, so they won't work unless you increase the number of tablets.

This list is just a very basic start. You will need to see your expert for a personalised plan, after a gold standard blood test is done, e.g. CMA intracellular vitamin test.

Flush your liver - Boost your hormones naturally
Hormones are the base of all your biochemistry, they assist all other bodily reactions and are vital to your immune system and your defence against disease.

A simple start; x2 tsp psyllium husk with ¾ glass of water on waking. You can buy it from Coles/Woollies or chemist.

If you respond badly to psyllium husk (funny tummy, coeliac), you can try;

Milk thistle (*iherb* is a good website, comes in tablet form) in the morning with breakfast.

Zinc - 40mg a day, take with breakfast
We don't have much in our soils in WA due to monoculture farming (nor manganese, magnesium, and other essential minerals, all listed on the WA agriculture department website). You can't produce hormones in your body without zinc, see picture at the end. Everyone needs to be on zinc (remember growth development/stimulation by hormones starts at 6 years of age on average).

Evidence shows that progesterone (in women) and thyroxine (women and men) support upper respiratory tone (open airways). Thus, less clenching, possibly grinding in sleep. Reference; Tarja Saaresranta 1, Olli Polo. Hormones and Breathing, Chest. 2002 Dec;122(6):2165-82. doi: 10.1378/chest.122.6.2165.

Evidence is very poor with measuring whether hormone therapy in men with sleep apnoea helps, as many other conditions will also occur, like obesity, high cholesterol. (Also the studies are only done on older men, i.e. >50yrs?).

Many younger men are experiencing fatigue, clenching, headaches, poor sleep. We know, poor sleep leads to lower testosterone. Being overweight significantly decreases testosterone. Thus, men need to lose weight before hormone therapy if over 50yrs (from one article that has low subject numbers?).

But wouldn't it be better to catch this before it becomes a chronic condition!!!?? Surely seeing an earlier pattern in younger men, will dramatically decrease the developing respiratory and cardiovascular risk. Thus, stop them becoming grossly overweight before they reach 40 - 50yrs of age.

Dr Dan Purser describes the benefits of normalising testosterone levels in men naturally (i.e. finding out the vitamin deficiencies responsible) to allow for weight reduction, reducing cardiovascular risk, optimising energy levels etc.

Reference: substack, Dr Dan Purser, 50+ Referenced Benefits Of Normalizing Testosterone Levels Naturally in MEN!

His online program (and in videos on Facebook), are extremely systematic and thorough.

Vit D - Is a hormone not a vitamin
How do you tell you get enough vit D? The basic rule of thumb is to have large surface area of skin to the sun (naked) for 10 min between 10am - 3pm. I.e. you need to have the larger surface areas of your body exposed to the sun. If you don't, you need the supplement. My favourite is; BioCeuticals D3 + K2 spray.

If you have a history of skin cancer, or basal cells, it is safer to take the supplement.

Magnesium
Important for muscle regulation, sleep, muscle cramps, helps with testosterone production (small amount in women, main hormone for men) and many other processes.

Vitamin C - 1000mg/day, take with breakfast
Helps you absorb zinc. Evidence to support immunity.

Sinus Irritation - Post nasal drip
A naturopathic chiropractic lecturer at a headache/migraine conference I attended in 2019, suggested for sinus issues take; three times the dosage of horseradish/garlic/vit C for 2 weeks. (Not to be taken as a preventor, but a stimulator of your immune system). Many of Leigh's clients have had good success with this when the Nasonex and other nose sprays that the ENT's recommend fail them.

CHAPTER 8

HORMONES

Hormones is a big topic and really important for your whole health.

Hormones are essential for maintaining your airways, especially at night when all your other muscles are relaxed... i.e. your clenching reflex.

Your sex hormones, Men (Testosterone and a small amount of Estrogen), and Women (Progesterone, Estrogen, DHEA, small amount of testosterone), are like the building blocks of your body. If they are not at an optimum, all your other bodies processes start to break down over time.

What erodes hormones, I hear you ask?
Stress - Biggest influencer, and now a big part of life since 2020, more than we have seen in a long time in human history.

Sugar - Particularly complex sugars (carbohydrates - pasta, rice), processed foods etc

Diesel - From cars and factories, especially sitting in cars on the freeway (google how much disease is created within a 200m radius next to freeways!! Very scary, the worst place to exercise next too).

Plastics - We constantly sit on and around plastics, and many of our kitchen surfaces have plastic compounds as part of the components. (Never mind the toxic glues used to glue those kitchen components together).

Therapists are starting to see people developing many more diseases, and at a much earlier age. I have seen an increase in clenching and grinding from all age groups, and particularly our younger generations from the increased scheduling of life and learning in front of screens.

Stats on jaw pain/TMD/Temporomandibular dysfunction says it is mostly 35-55 yr olds, 95% women, I feel this is outdated. I am treating a lot of teenagers and as young as 3 - 6 year olds with our neuro divergent personality adaptations to increased information absorption and high scheduling (stressful situations).

Evidence shows that Progesterone and Thyroxine are important for maintaining women's airways (i.e. Throat muscle tone) at night, when all your other muscles are relaxed and floppy. If progesterone and thyroxine are low, your airways become floppy and this is what increases the 'normal' clench reflex, so you start to over clench, and/or grind and/or snore/mouth breath. It is important to maximise your hormones to have the best airways at night and not create an oxygen debt, which will stress the whole body.

Reference: Tarja Saaresranta 1, Olli Polo. Hormones and Breathing, Chest. 2002 Dec;122(6):2165-82. doi: 10.1378/chest.122.6.2165.

For men testosterone is just as important, however the evidence and research is poor. The latest research, one article! Said that hormone replacement (of natural testosterone) may create floppier airways. The study was done on low numbers of subjects, was tested on men over 55yrs, so they already had co morbidities/conditions, that were not disclosed, neither was data on their weight, or BMI. No one has done a good, double blind study on young subjects, with normal weight/BMI to see what the base level is for airway management.

Lab Ranges for hormones
Lab ranges are vastly outdated, and not adapted to our sudden change in mental health, i.e. large amounts of stress due to 2020 event.

Hormone lab value levels from blood tests are based on 1000 white females. We have over 4 billion women on the planet. And different cultures need different amounts.

Also, if we take progesterone, it has 4 phases in our monthly cycle. You need to know which phase is the most important to look at depending on the age of the women. For example, 18yrs - 40yrs you should be looking at the luteal phase, not the total progesterone amount.

Dan Purser MD, (one the world's best in hormone information on safety and prescription levels) says that 18 - 40 year old women should be tested on day 21 of their cycle, and it should be above 30nMol/L.

And men, testosterone levels should be around 30 - 35 (the range is 10 - 35). Most men who see me in the clinic with jaw pain are around 11 - 25, this is an indication for testosterone cream prescription, if mental health is stable.

TIP: Dr Dan Pursers books measure in the American model - ng/mol, the Australian levels nMol/L, just use google conversion tables!

Most of Leigh's clients are in these low value ranges and all have jaw pain and headaches or migraines with many other symptoms or conditions.

How do you boost hormones naturally?
For Men - Google testosterone foods
For Women - Google progesterone foods, and eat more of these foods.

Liver
The Naturopaths I work with suggest flushing your liver. They endorse the benefits by saying it can boost your hormones if you flush your liver. (Remember, blood tests of liver function will only come up if 95% or more of your liver is dysfunctional. You don't want to wait that long to look after your liver. Make sure it is always healthy). This can be done with x2 tsp psyllium husk and ¾ glass of water, or milk thistle tablets, first thing in the morning. Or ask your naturopath for an individualised plan.

Zinc
We can't make hormones without this mineral.

The West Australian Agriculture department has a page dedicated to minerals in our soils. We are low in zinc, and deficient in Magnesium (important for testosterone making chains in our bodies) and manganese and many other trace elements. Doctors recommend 40 - 50 units, most multivitamins only have 10 - 20, so look on the bottle.

Vit D

Is a hormone, not a vitamin. The basic rule of thumb is to have large surface area of skin to the sun (naked) for 10 min between 10am - 3pm. I.e. you need to have the larger surface areas of your body exposed to the sun. If you don't, you need the supplement. My favourite is; BioCeuticals D3 + K2 spray.

If you have a history of skin cancer, or basal cells, it is safer to take the supplement.

Vitamin C

(Recommended dosage is 1000mg/day), take with breakfast. Helps you absorb zinc. Evidence to support immunity.

There is obviously much more to look at with your biochemistry and which systems are not functioning well. It is much better to have an individualised assessment and plan by a nutritionist/naturopath/nurse practitioner/ integrated GP.

This is a great starting point. No matter who my clients have seen they all start with this. So, I thought you might like to save some time.

Hormone Treatment (Bioidentical, not the pill)

This is based on my own research, please do your own, and make your own decisions. I have worked with hundreds of good doctors who admit to their level of training in this area, and many hundreds who have no training in this area. Be careful who you ask. As many doctors (especially in my 30 years of Endometriosis/IBS/Chronic fatigue I have seen a lot of specialist here in WA and in London) and as a referring therapist have come across many that have very limited professional development in this field, including specialists.

My reference is of someone who I consider to be a world leading expert, Dan Purser MD, *www.danpursermd.com.* Who has many easy-to-read/cheap books supporting safety and prescription (and we're not talking about the pill), and evidence-based research to back up his ideas in his books, podcasts and sub stack records. I greatly appreciate the nurse practitioners of Australia, who I find have a more thorough understanding of hormone assessment & therapy and its importance in whole health prevention and management.

Dan Purser MD, talks about bio identical hormones. How much safer they are than the pill and how much more effective, in his books, podcasts and sub stack.

For the last 4 years of practice (since 2019) in this field a majority of my client's have been assessed and managed with bioidentical hormones, instead of or alongside of; anti-depressants, Valium, steroids etc with a great reduction in symptoms, and a healing of their co morbidities.

In Dr Dan Pursers progesterone book, page 14 tells you that natural progesterone, P4, reduces your risk of breast cancer by 540% and all other cancers by 1000%.

You might know of it as Prometrium, the compounded form by a chemist in trouche form (gum substance that goes under your lip) is much cheaper, and according to Dr Dan Purser, more effective in absorption into the body than the tablet and cream form.

Ref: Cowan LD, Gordis L, et al. Breast cancer incidence in women with a history of progesterone deficiency. Am J Epidemiol. 1981.

Many doctors are not trained in bioidentical hormones, so they are prescribing two types of pills, or the Merina and a small pill, as they have found that the pill is one dose and cannot possibly address all the differences in females. The pill is only one dose. No other medication is one dose for 4 billion people. You need different amounts of hormones depending on your; age, co morbidities/conditions, and more importantly the stress/mental health.

Important to note: No one will prescribe you hormones if you are mentally unstable, i.e. not actively trying to manage your stress, internal voices/self-criticism etc. When you are highly stressed, no matter how much good biochemistry (vitamins, minerals, hormones) you put in your body, you will erode them straight away. Your therapist will be looking to see how you are managing your stress/mental health. You will have to be honest and share this information. Many clients are hesitant, and even paranoid to discuss their mental health. But your therapist needs to know about your whole health if they are going to be able to change your symptoms quickly and effectively.

Another great book all about hormones, especially for the younger generation, teaching them healthy habits around periods and how your period will tell you about your whole health, is called, Period Repair Manual by Lara Briden. It also details how the pill is not good for our bodies.

I love Dr Dan Pursers books on hormones, they are so good in letting you know of all the age-related diseases you will greatly reduce or stop, if you have optimum hormones. Like big reductions or no, cardiovascular disease (stroke, heart attack), osteoporosis, high cholesterol, weight gain, depression/anxiety, etc. Now that's what I want to hear when I see a doctor, what we need for normal health, what are normal levels, what else I will be preventing if I make an effort.

This is where taking responsibility becomes a big part of your new mindset. Hearing new information without allowing the triggering to block you, just taking it in as research.

Hormones – Biochemical Pathways

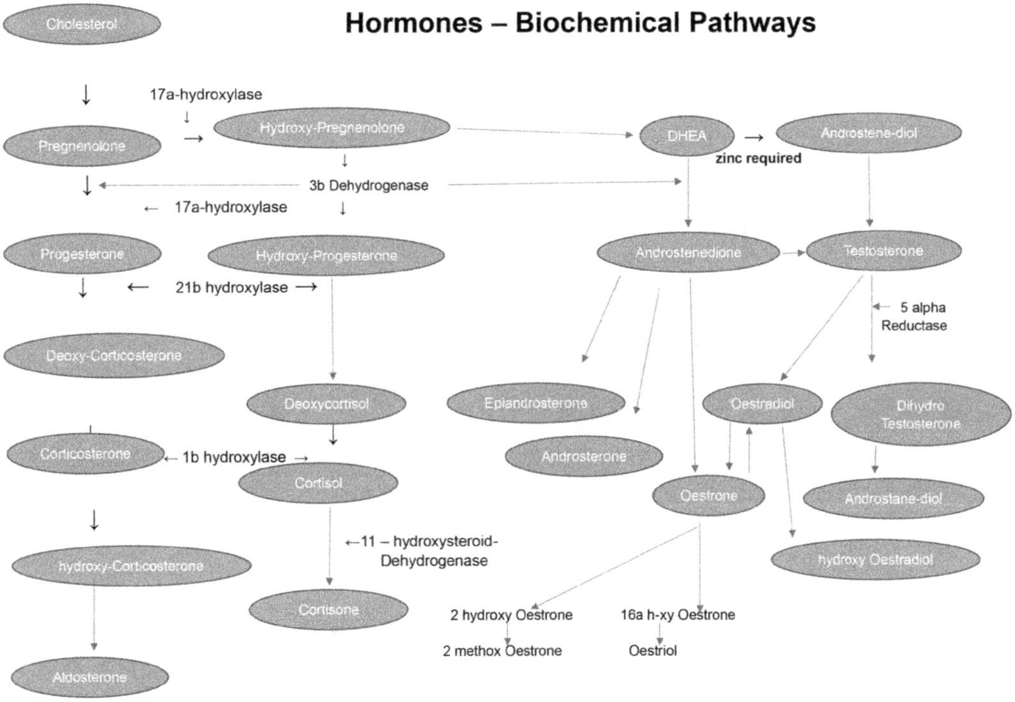

Cholesterol

17a-hydroxylase

Pregnenolone

Hydroxy-Pregnenolone

3b Dehydrogenase

17a-hydroxylase

Progesterone

Hydroxy-Progesterone

21b hydroxylase

Deoxy-Corticosterone

Deoxycortisol

Corticosterone

1b hydroxylase

Cortisol

11 – hydroxysteroid-Dehydrogenase

hydroxy-Corticosterone

Aldosterone

Cortisone

DHEA

zinc required

Androstene-diol

Testosterone

5 alpha Reductase

Dihydro Testosterone

Androstane-diol

hydroxy Oestradiol

Androstenedione

Oestradiol

Oestrone

Epiandrosterone

Androsterone

16a h-xy Oestrone

Oestriol

2 hydroxy Oestrone

2 methox Oestrone

47

CHAPTER 9

THYROID & INSULIN RESISTANCE
A big part of TMD, migraines and headaches

Have you had a complete thyroid panel done?

Low or high thyroid levels can lead to an increase in your clenching and grinding at night, as thyroxine is important for keeping your airways open at night when all your other muscles are relaxed. You can suffer with jaw click/clunk/pain, headaches, migraine, ear pressure/fluid/noise/pan.

If you have this condition, then you really need a better diet, and guess what, normal progesterone levels, will allow you to control this condition so much easier, i.e. you won't need as many medications. A lot of TMD/jaw pain/migraine clients have this condition.

There are 5 important pieces when it comes to the thyroid puzzle. TSH, FT4, FT3, Thyroid Antibodies and Reverse T3. Unfortunately, it isn't uncommon for only TSH to be tested... and if you are lucky, FT4. I encourage you to be your own health advocate and ask for a full thyroid panel to be tested.

Let me explain these in a bit more detail.

TSH stands for thyroid stimulating hormone. This basically tells us if your brain - the pituitary gland, specifically - is telling your thyroid to make thyroid hormone. If you are not getting enough of this signal, then you will not make sufficient levels of thyroid hormone (hypothyroidism). On the other hand, if you are getting a big signal, then you can make too much thyroid hormone (hyperthyroidism). From a functional perspective this should be between 1 and 2. Anything over two can indicate hypothyroidism.

When your thyroid gets the signal from your brain to make thyroid hormone, it makes FT4. However, this is the inactive form of thyroid hormone. That is not to say it is not important though. We need to have sufficient levels of the inactive thyroid hormone to be able to be converted to the active form, which is the FT3.

From a functional perspective, FT4 should be at least in the middle of the reference range, if not in the upper 3/4 of the range.

The process of converting FT4 to FT3 mostly takes place in the liver. It is the FT3 that should enter the cells and do the thyroid hormone job. If this conversion doesn't happen, then there can be hypothyroid symptoms occurring. Again, from a functional perspective, FT3 should be at least in the middle of the reference range, if not in the upper 3/4 of the range.

The other issue is that Reverse T3 can stop FT3 from entering the cell. The reason being, it binds to the receptor sites on the cells, essentially blocking the FT3 from being able to do so.

Reverse T3 is produced when we are stressed, so it is important to have stress management techniques in place. From a functional perspective this should be no higher than middle of the reference range. Any higher than that, and the FT3 will be impaired from getting into the cells and doing its job.

The last piece of the thyroid puzzle to test for are Thyroid Antibodies. If there is a known thyroid problem, it is beneficial to know if it is the autoimmune type. The autoimmune type of hypothyroidism is Hashimoto's thyroiditis. The autoimmune type of hyperthyroidism is Grave's disease.

Knowing exactly what is going on with each piece of the thyroid puzzle will give a much better guideline for further investigation and/or how to specifically tailor your treatment. **Permission/Credit: Jen Knutson, Naturopath/Nutritionist.**

Have you been tested for insulin resistance?
Insulin is another hormone. It is released by the pancreas. When you eat food, insulin is released so that cells know to open up and convert that food/sugar into energy. When you're resistant, your cells don't open up, and excess sugar sits in the blood. And you release more and more insulin trying to cope.

Most of these people don't have any symptoms, but it does lead to other health problems; headaches, jaw grinding/clenching, foggy head, fatigue, etc.

Multiple tests make the diagnosis, including and not limited to, bit of weight gain, BMI changes, above average blood pressure but not high, changes in blood sugar tests and fasting sugars, and cholesterol changes.

This is why a regular routine of movement/exercise is so important, and regular sex hormone testing. As normalisation of weight is more to do with hormones than exercise and diet as you get older, i.e. over 40 years. Most of the world's research on exercise is based on men. Most women over 40 years (not all) won't reduce weight easily with cardio exercise, often it makes them put on more weight. Doing 7- 5min of exercise, where you rest when you are breathless and get back into it when you feel more able and confident is more beneficial. No, there is not any research to support this yet, but you all know it.

From a habit point of view, you need to do exercise you love doing (don't force yourself to the gym), pick up outdoor activities you love, like/ walk/skip with dog at the beach, snorkelling, dancing (any style at home when no one is watching), social new age dance (drug free groups to live DJ's are all the rage), parkour, qi gong, Pilates, yoga, hiking, cycling etc

CHAPTER 10

AIRWAYS, SINUS & SALIVA GLANDS

Airways

Snoring is not an indication of sleep apnoea, for either men or women, according to the latest research.

The 3 main questions the sleep doctors/dentists are asking as an introduction for whether they need to investigate whether you have a sleep airway obstruction/apnoea, are:

1) Do you wake up feeling refreshed?
2) Do you sleep with your mouth open (i.e. drool on pillow, dry throat / lips? Or through your nose.
3) Do you sleep on your side / back / tummy.

Answering positively to 2 out of 3, indicates you need further investigation into whether you have sleep apnoea. I.e. a positive response means = don't feel refreshed on waking in the morning (even if you have children), sleep with your mouth open, sleep on your tummy or back.

Now we all know that if you sleep on your tummy, you will always have neck issues and no one will be able to fix that, and it dramatically blocks your airway. Sleeping on your back can lead to the tongue sliding back into your throat, during REM cycle sleep patterns and blocking your airway for some of the time you are asleep.

If you measure moderate to severe sleep apnoea, then you will need an appliance, either CPAP or a mandibular advancement splint.

If you have just a regular splint, without having the sleep study test, you could be reducing your airway further, so make sure you have been checked out for the possibility of airway reduction, before your dentist makes a general splint (more about types of splints in the next chapter).

The sleep studies that can be done at home, usually rented out by the chemists according to the research is not effective enough, and just a start point to say you need to pay the money and do the sleep in the sleep clinic over night. So you may as well just go straight there.

Reduced airways can show up as headaches/migraines/fatigue/brain fog/heart attacks etc, so you need to check it out, with a proper sleep doctor at their lab.

Obviously, it will not replicate a normal night's sleep like at home, but it is the best situation we have to test you. The iPhone wrist watches/amazon oximeter's/iPhone apps are not accurate enough...yet!!! (watch this space).

Best ways to keep a good airway at night;

1) Lose weight, most of us know when we are overweight, it's quite logical, the basic google BMI tests will give you an indication. Also look at your throat and see if there is extra fat around your throat, if there is, you need to reduce your bad fats and sugars +++++/quickly.

   So healthy diet, no sugar, good fats, no processed food, no additives.

2) Test your sex hormone levels, for women the important one is progesterone, as this allows pharyngeal muscles to stay toned to protect your airway (when all other muscles are relaxed), just as testosterone does for men. Even a small drop in either can be enough to make your throat muscles floppy and reduce your airways. I see quick changes within 3 - 6 months of taking bio identical hormones. Obviously, a follow up test by the sleep doctors after losing weight, good diet, low to no alcohol/drugs, low stress, to make sure you don't need the splint after making these changes.

3) Don't lie on your tummy. Changing this is habit is hard, but possible. Take 6 weeks, for the first 2 weeks put a pillow under one knee to wedge you over a little, every 2 weeks add another pillow until you are wedged onto your side. Or use one of those long sausage shaped pregnancy pillows to hug and put between your knees to keep you on your side. This is really important and will reduce severe neck later in life.

4) Reduce alcohol/drug intake. If using alcohol try for Fri - Sun, only 1-3 glasses. Remember AA (alcoholics

anonymous) and Al-anon (for friends and family of addicts) are great free services for food/drug/alcohol addiction, just google for your closest group meeting. If you are not sure you are addicted, the definition is not the frequency of the activity, but the inability to stop, once you start that product.

Sinus

A lot of Leigh's clients are referred by ENT's with recurrent sinus infections, irritations, rhinitis, fluid feeling in ears, dripping ears that aren't dripping, ears that do drip and have no source, post nasal drip.

A lot of these issues resolve with jaw physio treatment and the extra information in this book, like better diet, less/no sugar, more meat and veggies (less pasta, rice, gluten, dairy), and vitamin supplements, see the other chapters on diet and vitamins.

Most clients are prescribed Nasonex by the ENT's and other variations of medications. The clients Leigh sees do not respond to these prescriptions. So, I have other options that my clients have endorsed. They will do no harm anyway.

These remedies are from naturopath's and biochemists.

Honey

Get your honey from your local bee keeper in your suburb (not the honey on the shelf from the shops, it is usually from NSW).

⅛ tsp x3 - 4/day for a month. Whether it's in warm water, smoothies, however you like it.

Garlic / Horseradish / Vit C

It comes in one tablet.

x3 times the dosage for 2 weeks and then stop taking it. Reassess your symptoms for 2 weeks, if still mucus/snot, re do for another 2 weeks.

This is not a preventor medication, it is used to wake up your immune system and dry out the sinus's.

Other PhD Biologist. Anthropologist, Herbalist I follow is Nicole Appelian's remedies.
https://nicolesapothecary.com/products/yarrow-tincture

And Leigh's treatments often shift a lot of mucus. Some clients are able to just blow their nose, others have had fluid come out of their ears and nose for 1-3 days, all reviewed by ENT's as normal for these conditions, and wonderful because the ENT's wont have to clear it out with surgery.

CHAPTER 11

MOUTH SPLINTS (NIGHT OCCLUSAL SPLINTS), BRUXISM & SLEEP HYGIENE

Bruxism
Is the grinding or gnashing of the teeth for no apparent reason during the daytime, usually semi-voluntary movement of the lower jaw. Grinding is usually on your front teeth and will show signs of wear.

Different to Sleep Bruxism - An involuntary motor activity during sleep associated with tooth grinding and often leads to problems with the jaw, neck and headaches.

Clenching - Everyone does it at night in their sleep and does not show wear on your teeth!!! When it increases, it becomes a problem (pathology). It is the meeting of the back teeth, in different parts of your sleep cycle, to when you could possibly grind your teeth. Is often done all day long with increased stress or on the start of a new activity. You don't have to clench down hard to start causing problems and over activity of your power muscles (Masseter muscles).

The Masseter muscles over power the endurance muscles and change the activation pattern of your jaw muscles. Just like the rest of the body, your deepest muscles should fire first, then the next layer, then the next layer. By clenching you are stopping your deep endurance muscles from working first and allowing just your top layer of muscles (the power muscles) to work all the time. They get tired and fatigue and cause a poor pattern of jaw opening and closing, causing pain and dysfunction. Leigh has some great "jaw Pilates" exercises to reboot your muscles to allow your jaw to open and close properly and reduce the pain and clicking and locking. See her online course at *https://www.jawphysio.com.au/diy-jawphysio-courses*

Normal Sleep - Duration is between 6 to 9 hours over a 24 hr circadian rhythm. Non REM sleep is 75-80% of your sleep and associated with body movement and sleep bruxism. (Kato et al 2003a) 74% of cases this bruxism occurs with clients sleeping on their backs, the same position which sleep apnoea clients sleep in. (Lavigne et al 2005a).

Best sleep position is on your side, with knees bent, small pillow or sock between your knees to support your lower back, arm crossed to stop you rolling forwards onto your chest (no hands under your jaw or head). Tilt the pillow down towards your shoulder so that you can tuck your chin in and maintain the best airway. If your pillow is against the bed head you often end up extending/tilting your head up, closing off your airway, which will lead to more clenching.

Splint Treatment
If you have jaw pain and headaches with no sleeping disturbance, see a Specialised Dentist or Oral-facial doctor for an occlusion splint (night guard). The normal dentists splints are designed to protect your teeth from cracking with clenching and grinding, and are fine if you have no jaw/head pain.

If you have jaw/head pain and clenching/grinding you will need a specialist dentist splint.

Most commonly clients are referred onto expert night occlusion splint (like a mouth guard) dentists/specialists who have also have training in sleep/respiratory medicine. If you have a restriction of airways and the wrong splint is made (i.e. reduces your airways further) you could become quite ill. Ask our team for the correct referral. Not all therapists who make splints have extensive training.

Occlusion Splints
Are much better as a lower jaw appliance (if you have TMJ symptoms/headaches or scan changes), they come as either a:
- decompressive splint, or neutral splint.

The acrylic splints take longer to mould, however they are more comfortable and sit lower in the mouth.

Proxy splints are cheaper/quicker to mould, however they are bulkier and affect the tongue position in the mouth, which we know will then affect sleeping (i.e. oxygen uptake or degree of bruxism).

The top occlusal splint only protect you from cracking your teeth, and are often the only training most dentists have. You have to have extra training/courses to know when to use the lower splints. The dental degree only trains dentists in the upper splint. There is evidence that night splints help. However no overwhelming evidence to support why upper splints only protect teeth, and lower splints work better if you have jaw joint, and or headaches/migraines involved with your symptoms.

Sleep disturbance = snoring, tired in the day, partner reports teeth/jaw noises. See a sleep study clinic. Mandibular advancement devices can be made, or CPAP therapy (continuous positive airway pressure device).

Most of Leigh's clients say they are able to wean off their splints if they take on all the options in this book, good diet, hormones, exercise, hobbies, work life balance, health boundaries in relationships, with a review at their dentist to make sure their teeth are in good condition.

Sleep Hygiene
Most of my clients are insomniacs, don't sleep well or long, or are constantly wake.

Did you know depression is a sleep disorder.

3am is the clenching/bruxism hour, and also the liver hour. Which makes sense as most of my clients are low in their sex hormones. If the sex hormones are low, it means they are not breaking down effectively and building up in your liver, rather than your blood stream. So the liver has to work harder, and often you are hotter at this time, whilst the liver is over worked.

Really important to see an integrated GP or nurse practitioner who is experienced at looking at hormones. Go and get a blood test for your sex hormones, women (progesterone, DHEA, estrogen, testosterone), men (testosterone, estrogen). See the hormone chapter for more information on this topic.

Ok so what is sleep hygiene?
It's not just getting up at the same time and going to bed at the same time. It is choosing 5-10 things to do, to let your brain work out, it needs to wind down and relax to allow for dreaming. Remember as a child, your mum fed you, bathed you, read you a story, tucked you into bed, maybe sung to you, put your night light on and told you - you were loved and safe.

Well from psychology, that little child, always stays with us, in our unconscious, and it needs to be loved, made safe and looked after!

The cognitive behaviour therapy with psychologists have treatment for sleep, and their course goes for 6 weeks. Here are some tips to get you started.

Pick some things off your joy list (ahhhh now what's an effing joy list I hear you say? Suffice to say, stuff that is not to do with work or caring for other humans).

So, your list might look like this.

- Finish screen time 1-2 hrs before bed!!! (eeeecckk). Shower/bath (last 2 minutes of shower is good to turn to all cold, has amazing results for better sleep), moisturise, water (no alcohol, it is a big stimulant for clenching, try to just have alcohol Fri-Sun).
- Light a candle.
- Pick a hobby to look over (try not to be on a screen for this).
- Walk around the block or house. In the old days you would walk around the farm with your dog at sunset and do a perimeter walk to make sure the land/animals/ pastures were ok.
- So in modern society we need to make sure you see the neighbours settling in, wave and smile and let your unconscious know, others know you are home and

to watch out for you. Say goodnight to your garden, appreciate the stars/moon. Check all the windows and doors are locked.

- Meditate or reflect on your day and all the nice things you did for others or how it made them feel when you helped others, i.e. gratitude diary. This is VERY important, do not reflect on your problems or inconveniences.

- Over emphasis on the good things, and your ability to try to be nice/happy/helpful, the more you do it, the more it comes back to you.

- You try and look at other perspectives in a friction moment of the day, put your "big adult pants" on and think, how could I have acted differently for that moment to not be so negative, or not for me to react so intensely.

- Psychology/religion/spirituality/neuroscience we know you can burn new neural pathways this way and it is highly effective in putting you on the path to higher emotions (satisfaction, happiness, contentment, bliss, love), but it needs to be trained, and you need to discipline yourself to do it every night. With big families you can talk about it around the dinner table, including kids from 3 yrs and older.

CHAPTER 12

PELVIC FLOOR & LOWER BACK PAIN

Many of my clients also suffer with lower back pain, and or pelvic floor pain.

Chronic lower back pain, has undergone a lot of serious study in the physio and chiro world, exploring what is generating the pain. Whether it be compressed (squished) nerves or swollen disc's. Most of the worlds top Physio's will tell you that chronic lower back pain is more related to how your brain interprets your pain, than the actual physical structures being the cause. Just like any other chronic pain, it takes at least x10 things to change, to change your chronic pain. So, a big part of recovery is working on your brain. You get to decide how to learn about your brain, whether its with a pain clinic with medication and pacing activities and functional movement classes, or with psychologist/psychotherapist, counsellor, spiritual healer, or faith based. No one technique works for everyone, as we all have different interpretations of our childhood, cultural and social influences, learning styles and much more.

I do find however, the topic of pelvic floor dysfunction, still quite hidden or taboo even in the West. A lot of my jaw, migraine clients will have some sort of pelvic floor dysfunction, whether it be dryness, itchy/candida, pain, odd sensations, pins and needles, pain with doing a wee or poo, or some sort of wee or poo leakage, irritation / redness to tearing of skin and muscle with sex or exercise. Over tightness of the pelvic floor, so unable to insert a tampon, pain with exercise and sex. Or too loose pelvic floor, feeling the pelvic floor starting to fall down and come outside of the body. No orgasm with self-stimulation or with a partner. All of which are not normal.

The women's health physio's do an absolute wonderful job at assessing where the issue is coming from. Whether it is muscle, nerve, or central nervous system. If you are a chronic pain person, you are more than likely going to have pelvic floor problems, as the whole nervous system, from the brain, down the spine, to the pelvic floor, is one continuous structure. This over sensitisation often creates pain, pins and needles, or numbness in the pelvic floor. Muscle retraining and nerve pacifying (whether with drugs, or tens machine, or Kegel type tools) often fail this type of client.

Having suffered severe endometriosis, my central sensitisation and pelvic floor issues started at the age of 6. I remember having x2-3 issues a year of burning pain for a week until I was 14 years old, where my pelvic pain was continuous with the start of my periods. I didn't realise it was so bad, as it was always there, until gynaecologists assessed me, and I would haemorrhage for 2-3 days after assessments. I had 4 GP's tell me the quicker I got pregnant the better from the age of 14. Never mind the gynaecologists that didn't believe me that I couldn't insert a tampon at age 14, and forced one in me, even though I was screaming at the top of my lungs!!! Another so called women's health GP advised me to 'just have affairs' when finding out I was single at age 34, despite all my pain in my pelvic floor. I found this thoughtless and stupid.

I have had a lot of traumatic experiences with specialists, and unfortunately, I hear similar stories at least once a month from my clients. Thank goodness, our specialists are learning that vulva vestibulitis and other similar conditions are not due to 'naughty' or 'difficult' women.

Its also not something any of us want to talk about. So, I thought I would be brave and describe some of the things that I experienced.

The women's health physio's reduced my central pain (spinal cord and pelvic floor pain) 25-50%, the drugs did absolutely nothing, and I stopped going to gynaecologists, as every single visit (I visited over 4 different ones in Perth) resulted in severe pain, haemorrhaging and flare up of all body pain for weeks after.

What changed my pain forever, 6 years ago, was bio

identical hormones, learning about inner child, and going through psychotherapy, mind discipline with meditation, setting of boundaries around my family. This took 3 - 4 years of weekly homework, x1 - 2 week long retreat courses per year, monthly therapy. But what a game changer. I was at the stage where I couldn't sit or stand for more than 2 hours a day. I slept for 3 days and nights, so that I could work for 4 days and repeated this cycle for 10 years. I was ready to die.

You do need to be careful who you can trust with this information, as many doctors, even specialists have no understanding, sympathy, or training in this area. I find the women's health physio's, endocrinologists and psychologists/psychotherapists much better trained in this area and know the doctors who are experienced and who to trust. And unfortunately, when I visit the international oral medicine lectures, pelvic pain is often brought up as a common co morbidity, but most of the male doctors and dentist/periodontists in the lectures, giggle nervously and admit they don't feel confident in talking about it with their clients. So, the whole health, whole body picture is often missed.

Keep searching ladies. You do not need to put up with pain, there are good therapists and doctors out there, who can guide you. Make sure you do your research.

CHAPTER 13

MEDICATIONS, BOTOX & SURGERY

If you can't change your triggers; diet, alcohol intake, coffee intake, life-work balance, reduce chores (get a cleaner, order household stapes/food online, grow your own veggies/fruit trees), get hobbies, be around people who nourish you. Then you can see your doctor for prescriptions. These are some top tips your GP might not know about.

I understand, sometimes, to be able to get healthy, you need to take some pills to get you on track. But write a contract with yourself and have a plan on the baby steps you will take to detox your life of bad habits, most of us know them.

You no longer have an excuse that you don't know what a healthy diet is with the internet around. The very least, if you do no processed foods, no fizzy drinks and put x4 - 6 cups of veggies into your day, you are more than on your way.

Have an accountability person who you chat with once a month for your plan - friend or GP for example.

Steroids - Prednisolone
A handy alternative if your TMD/Jaw Pain is over 8/10 and not settling with treatment and anti inflammatories after 2-6 weeks. Usually 25mg is prescribed for 3-5 days with review. This dosage is small, similar to a dosage for bee stings and asthma attacks. Contraindications are recent psychotic attack, or recent cardiac event. Low to no risk of Cushon's disease as its only for 3 days.

Botox for jaw pain, has 30% effective rate, determined by the latest research, to help with bruxism (over clenching and grinding). I see so many clients who have had it into their masseter muscles, and these muscles start to weaken, the facial muscles then move or droop because the continual use of Botox is changing the way the musculature work around the face and jaw.

And I see a lot of side effects with Botox, jaw joint erosion, from poor motor pattern recruitment, locked jaws from Botox'ing the incorrect muscles from poor assessment.

Clients often say the first dose of Botox works well, then the body gets used to it and is no longer as effective for future dosages. Its expensive at $600-$1000 per dosage. Cheaper dosages means the Botox is being diluted with saline and will not be effective.

Use it if you have tried everything else and you are in a lot of pain. It is a last resort, to give you time to determine your triggers in life.

Botox for migraines - much higher success rate. It works well for a lot of people.

However, I think it is important to find the source. Many psychologists I treat, comment that migraines are related to listening to the critical voice in your head, over scheduling, listing to the chaos in your brain. There is a lot more brain evolution work related to this condition, see more in the Quantum physics and the brain chapter.

Autoimmune Conditions
LDN - Low dose naltrexone has become an effective alternative to some of the very toxic rheumatology drugs. A good rheumatologist will be open to discussing alternatives.

Used for and not limited to; Ankylosing spondylitis, Chronic fatigue syndrome, Endometriosis, Hashimoto's, Luus, Parkinson's disease, Rheumatoid Arthritis, Chrones disease, Coeliac disease, Alzheimer's disease, Inflammatory bowel disease, multiple sclerosis, Psoriasis, Sarcoidosis, Ulcerative colitis... any condition that may be associated with inflammation.

It has virtually no side effects. It requires a titrate dose, i.e. slow increase over a few weeks, so you need someone who knows what they are doing.

Metformin is being used for insulin resistance and diabetes. Metformin is used to treat high blood sugar levels that are caused by a type of diabetes mellitus or sugar diabetes called type 2 diabetes. With this type of diabetes, insulin produced by the pancreas is not able to get sugar into the cells of the body where it can work properly.

Is Metformin being discontinued?
Out of an abundance of caution, we extended the recall to all lots of metformin hydrochloride extended-release tablets in the US. Apotex stopped selling this product in the U.S. in February 2019, and there remains only limited product on the market.

Is there a good substitute for metformin?
Three new treatments for type 2 diabetes have been recommended by NICE, for patients who cannot use metformin, sulfonylurea or pioglitazone. The treatments are also suitable for patients who are not controlling their blood glucose levels with diet and exercise alone, to manage their condition.

Side effects of medications
Many medications have side effects, which can cause; headaches, dizziness and tinnitus. The information is on the information paper/brochure inside the packet, or you can google them. From your run of the mill anti inflammatory to the potent rheumatology and cholesterol drugs.

As we get older, it is standard procedure for your GP to prescribe you more medications, which have greater risk of side effects and interfering with each other, creating more issues, where more medications are prescribed. Seems like a bit of a circle. This isn't just my opinion, but that of Dr Dan Purser. He has many blogs, Facebook posts, substack evidenced based lectures on how to get whole health, without using as many strong medications that interact with other organs.

I highly recommend his very affordable books and information from his website *www.danpursermd.com*

CHAPTER 14

POSITIVE PARENTING

There are lots of fabulous courses with many more examples. I have just chosen some simple ideas that have worked well for my clients, that are easy to remember and hopefully easy to action. Please do your own research and use what works for your family.

Start a family dinner meeting about these ideas.

First Rule - Never speak in anger to another person. Particularly family members.

When you start to feel angry, you say to the other person.

'I am feeling triggered, I need to go away and think about what is triggering me and I will come back when I can discuss this calmly or as an adult.'

(Even if it's the other persons fault).

Anger can take 5min to 3 days to dissolve and allow you to look at all the perspectives of the discussion. (Perspectives; yours, theirs, reality, how you were brought up, and many other angles, at least 12!). Make sure you mark a time in your diary/phone to come back to that person and discuss the issue. If you don't you are just ignoring your trigger and it will get much bigger, and you will stress about it.

The trick is to set your boundary, not make them see how much of a victim they made you feel like. E.g. please don't put me down in a joke, its mean and you're narcissistic, and always so bitchy around me. This is victim mode. A good boundary sounds like, you hurt my feelings, I would like you to be an active listener, please increase your support around me, and only give me positive feedback. If you can't then please don't say anything.

Second Rule - How to communicate with each other in a trigger moment.

When someone brings up a problem, it is helpful and adult to say;

'So what I'm hearing is that...' and repeat what the person said.

This allows both people to hear out loud what is proposed, as your internal thoughts can be illogical or a bit mixed up.

That gives the first person a chance to say, 'yes that's right', Or

'No I said', the second person keeps repeating until they both hear the same thing.

Or

The first person says 'oh don't worry, that's not as bad as I thought now I've heard it out loud.'

Then the second person has a chance to think about the idea, and say, well I agree with the first part, but I can't do the second, but I can do something else, is this helpful?

The first person repeats the process above and says, 'So I heard you say...' And repeats the second persons answers.

Neither party has to agree, but you have to both honour each other's thoughts/feelings and that you heard correctly, in a calm manner. You then keep discussing until both parties get what they want (neither has to compromise).

If you can't come to an arrangement, then you arrange to discuss the topic in a week or a month, until you both agree on an arrangement that works for both parties.

Stephen R. Covey (famous for his book, The 7 habits of highly effective people), disagrees with this technique, and seeks you to be an active listener, seek to understand first, so he gets you to ask the person questions until you both understand, showing a sense of empathy and understanding and time of what the person is saying. I agree with this. However, most of my clients are so tired and overscheduled, I find the above technique better at slowing both parties down, so you have time to listen. Which is a big skill. Most people will guess first, or have judgement triggers as you talk.

It takes practice to just listen.

Third Rule - Children only need to hear 3 things; I love you, you're safe, I see how hard you are trying/working.

This is about how to talk to children and not triggering, getting angry, frustrated and sounding like a teenager yourself!!

The Psychologists tell us children will ask the same question 7 times up to the age of 14. It is how their brain grows and is trying to link the synapses.

Accept this as a growing issue, it is not them being rude/ cheeky/disbelieving.

First give the child a kind/neutral instruction, with 2 choices that are toward the goal you wish. (Make sure your tone of voice is low and calm and a little bit quiet).

This allows them to feel a sense of self and power with the choices.

DO NOT justify this instruction, do not over explain.

If they can't remember, or constantly say 'why?', answer their questions with:

'I love you', or 'you're safe', or 'I can see how hard you are trying/working.'

This allows them to think through the original question and makes them problem solve and self soothe what you are saying. You need to give them a chance to work it out for themselves.

(Children under 3-4 yrs you will have to give more simple instructions and perhaps repeat yourself).

Example:
Parent - Put your shoes on so we can go to swimming lessons, if you don't, we will be staying home with no Wi-Fi.

Child - Tantrum/distracted - Child misses swimming and

consequence is enacted without explanation nor eruption from parent. Child will ask why we didn't go to swimming. Answer with 'I love you' (not, I told you what would happen if you didn't put your shoes on).

Or

Child – Why?

Parent – I love you

Child – Why

Parent – You're safe

Child – Why are you speaking like that?

Parent – I love you

(And repeat until the child makes a decision. You are going to accept that you will be late and miss some activities in the first 2 - 4wks of starting this training). The parents are always so surprised how quickly the children catch on, as it is a calm tone of voice, and there is no eruption of anger or frustration, and they are aware they made the choice, and it was their consequence, not a yelling parent as the outcome.

If you as the parent feels like erupting and are very angry and can't do the 3 sentences, put your 'adult pants' on and own up. I am feeling angry/triggered, I don't want to speak to you angry, I'm going to think about this and come back and discuss it when I'm not angry.'

You're modelling that adults are not perfect, but you don't have to be your emotions/feelings, you can stop and relax and think about when you first felt this emotion and see what memory comes up for you as a child. And recognise the family templating from your parents, and how upset you got over a situation as a child. That you are not a child now, as an adult, you have processes, experience, capacity to deal with stressful situations and can apply models of behaviour to adapt to stress, without resorting to childish behaviour - angry/shouting/over explaining.

It takes practice of course, and own up, when you get it wrong. Your kids will love you for it. All the adults in the house must do the same words, and it works really quickly. My clients rave about this way of talking in the household.

It can be applied at work, obviously instead of saying 'I love you', you can say; 'you are loved', 'I love your work', 'thank you for thinking of me', etc Adapt it to your adult world.

Most importantly you learn that triggering is a learning experience, you are not failing/or not coping, you are learning, which is lifelong.

Learning about 'inner child' work is great for this. As you stop and think about the first time you felt a negative emotion, and then see how this event is driving you as an adult, when someone makes you feel that emotion again. Classically, how we feel around authority figures, bosses, government ideals (rates, speeding fines etc), all the things that make us feel powerless. But you don't have to feel powerless.

There are many more transformation processes to go through with a therapist to change this childhood trigger. Get reading about philosophy/psychology/spirituality and find out why your parents and the 10 parents behind them said the things they said, and how you are going to do things differently (not opposite, as this creates the same trauma/negative emotion).

There are many other ways to positively parent, but this is my favourite, as it is simple to remember and applies to any age.

CHAPTER 15

QUANTUM PHYSICS OR BRAIN EVOLUTION

"All of the Body is in the Mind. Only part of the mind is in the body." Credit *https://www.freedomfromchronicpain.com/* lecture series.

All the body is in the mind - the brain controls and gets feedback information on all the bodily functions, from chemical reactions to muscle contractions etc.

Only part of the mind is in the body - we know we only use around 5% of our brain for our daily life. Leaving us so much more room for other processes, e.g. mindfulness, meditation, manifestation of our future (imagining how we would like our lives to be - hope, daydreaming), and to look at the past (wisdom/knowledge and context of what works for us, what is our greatest joy and greatest good for our future selves).

Quantum physics has now proven that it is the same as spirituality (medicine calls it psycho-social aspects). We used to think that science and spirituality are separate. Science has now shown it is the same thing. In the simplest example, science has measured the atom precisely. The atom has been measured to be 99.9% space/energy and 0.01% mass. Our bodies are made up of millions of trillions of atoms. So, our bodies, our skin sack! is only 0.01% mass, the rest of us is space (otherwise known as energy). So, we can now see that our lives and how we integrate into reality is mostly energy. We can only change energy with our consciousness/our mind (our energy generator).

The mind is not the brain, as scientists still haven't found where our soul/consciousness/personality sits in the brain. Our consciousness is energy. Energy is infinite and according to Einstein cannot be created nor destroyed, just transformed. So, our mind is there to be awakened/transformed.

To transform you have to look at the beforehand (past) as well as manifest your greatest good for your future self.

To not think of the beforehand, alongside the future betterment of humankind is counterproductive.

Ancient cultures saw the complete body. Not just the skin sack and its symptoms that the medical profession looks at now.

To heal the body, we must also incorporate the mind and the context of the person. Context includes present, past and future.

More helpful to look at now. If the person has evolved their mind with mindfulness and meditation and asks for guidance, you can heal by going through the past and looking at the future.

Future is the persons feelings of how they want to be, and we know that manifests in reality.

Past is the persons subconscious, dreams, the collective consciousness, the interconnectedness of life and templating from parents in childhood (a structure in which to understand the world/reality).

To change your past (which is part of all of humankind), we have to go back to the past.

I.e. Quantum physic's. Time is not linear, but a moebius loop - infinite loop.

So basic steps. Where you have pain, is maybe just more dense matter. i.e. atoms oscillating closer together. So, visualise and feel the space between your atoms in that part of your body. Feel them further apart - more space. Not only feel lighter in that area but see a bright white/golden light in that area, that gets brighter as the space becomes less dense and thus the light becomes lighter. Thus the lighter light.

Pain/symptoms are transformed into nothing - quite literally much less dense atoms, more space and thus nearly nothing for the brain to register as pain/symptoms.

Outer mind = human concerns, desires

↓ healthy - water/organic food	↑ alcohol/pollution
↓ mindfulness, meditation	↑ rushing
↓ kindness	↑ consumer drive/desires
↓ pausing/stillness	

Inner mind = interconnected consciousness of the planet

The psychologists tell us that 97% of the western world is stuck in co dependence. And most of us have never had any training in positive mind work/positive parenting/or counselling for ourselves. To be more successful, you need to find out what triggers in yourself are triggering others around you, even if you think you are not dysfunctional. It is about taking responsibility for everything in your life. If anything bad happens, you are the only one who is always there, you are the recurring factor. So even if bad stuff happens, and you didn't instigate it, find out how reality works as to why you keep getting involved or shown bad stuff.

I absolutely love the free you tube book - Zero Limits, that describes these phenomena and how to change your reality for the greater good. It is not based on any religion or faith, and even says you don't need psychology to change your life. It is based on a Hawaiian philosophy and is life changing. I practice it every day, however I also like the psychology teachings, as you find out why you have that little voice in your head telling you that you're not good enough...etc (its called the critical parent voice), or why I keep running victimhood scenario's through my head (like why did that person talk to me like that, or why did that guy cut me off in traffic).

I really love the psychotherapy work with "inner child". It makes so much sense, where to send that self-love, when you find out the reason for being on the planet (is not 42, as the hitchhiker to the galaxy book proposes!!), but to fill yourself full of love. That is your joy list Then the second part to being on the planet, is to be of service to humanity. These 2 tenants are in every religion, faith, psychology. But you can't help others if you are empty.

How do you know if you are empty, your body displays pain/discomfort. The body doesn't have language, its language is pain, and it is letting you know, you need to check in with your soul/little child/personality/heart and scan your body for "what is wrong" or ask your body "what do you need?". It will tell you. But you need to get quiet and sit still for a while with your eyes closed. Your body will answer you with a memory or a symbol/colour.

You intuition is your strongest healer. Research is showing that precognition, is not actually a magical thing, your body knows what is wrong, and then the neuro science is really cool, it sends a little "intuition thought", which is actually your body saying, you need to fix this. The art is listening more often. You can't do this if you are rushing, empty, and forgetting to check in with yourself every 30min to see if you need the basic self care = self love = water/food/rest/toilet/move-stretch.

This is actually the start of therapy/counselling/psychology/spirituality/faith.

You start with this self care scan = ...do I need water/food/rest/bathroom/move-stretch. This scan should be done every 30min!!!

It is so important we start discussing these ideas with our children. The easiest way I see it is when they cry or lose their patience. This happens often as their brain is growing and they have no language to ask why it feels funny to have feelings or the change in energy - frustration, anger, increase in body temp with anger, decrease in body temp with fatigue.

Cry and outbursts need to be coupled with pausing. No matter where you are or what chores you think you need to get done.

That child needs to be told 'you're safe/, 'I'm here for you', 'I love you', 'you're safe', 'I'm here for you', 'I will stay with you whilst you ride this out'

Even from the age of 2. These principles should be talked about;

1) You are not your feelings, you can just watch them, instead of acting on them.

2) You are not all of your thoughts. If it's not a nice thought, pick another one that is efficient for a life of loving kindness.

3) You are human = imperfect. Its ok not to know the solution for every problem. Life is about loving the imperfections in yourself and in others. When we have an interaction with another human where it is awkward or tense, this is called a friction point. And it is how we grow and evolve. We need to start to like these 'friction points', as this is when we get to change and learn.

4) You can just sit quietly with your feelings and thoughts and just watch them. You do not need to act on those negative feelings or be in the middle of them, getting caught up in messy thoughts and feelings. Just sit back and go, oh that's interesting, I'm feeling... angry/frustrated/etc and just watch that feeling.

   Once it dissipates a bit, see if you can see the flip side to the thoughts/feelings that are making you angry/frustrated and once a positive feeling is found, then you can act on those emotions. And your life will be filled with more positive interactions.

5) It is really good to day dream, this only happens when you take time to sit still and do nothing. (So it is really important for parents to strictly limit screen time on social media and playing games. I.e. 10 - 30 min /day. There is a lot of evidence out there to show just how harmful social media is to the developing brain and adult brains). Being bored is really important for young peoples development, as it allows creativity to appear.

6) It is ok to surrender and let go of thoughts of friction and resistance and breathe.

The solution comes quicker from the "inner mind" when the outer mind just lets go/surrenders.

Joy List

Life is not about paying the mortgage and working (your job should take up 40% of your mental capacity! Say the psychologists and financial planners). If you are lucky you are working in a job you love. And if you are really enlightened you have managed to take something off your joy list and make it your job. Even the "Barefoot Investor" talks about this.

So firstly, why are you on the planet,? no idea! Well ask a kid, like I did the other day, and his immediate answer was;

"To have fun!" yes joy, self love, self nurturing. This is the first tenant of all psychology, philosophy, religion, spirituality.

Most people skip to the second tenant and forget the first - "to be of service to humanity." Well, you can't help anyone, if you are running on empty. Most mums I treat are more than empty, they are feeling like they have been run over several times.

How do you remember how to have fun and show your "inner child" how to have fun. Well, you can start with a vision board. I use the wardrobe door, and I have cut pictures out of magazines or printed them off the computer of all the things I love (places to travel to, pets, friends, gardens, architecture, textiles, flowers, money, motorbikes, ocean, sunshine, candles, etc). Then every time you walk past that board in the morning, it reminds you to put at least one of those things into your day.

Make sure you are filling up your day with your love, then you might one day have some energy for others. When you put everyone ahead of yourself, you burn out, get really sick, and then your kids get sick too. Start to think why the level of autism and ADHD has increased in the last 20 years. If you don't know, kids 20 years ago were diagnosed at 1 in 20. In the next 20 years it is predicted that 1 in 3 will be diagnosed on the ADHD spectrum, and not just from lack of knowing how to diagnose, its more to do with the amount of information people are being expected to hold in one day, the stress of high scheduling (coping with running a household and working and being a taxi driver etc). It has really stretched our brains, and we are not coping. So, more disorders are occurring.

So with that joy list, you start to realise how important it is to get a work - life balance!!!! The world health organisation said that women should only work 6hrs a day (as we have 35% less body muscle mass/strength, on average), and men should work no more than 8 hrs a day. To stay well men and women should only work 18 hrs a week. Most people do a heap more. The latest statistics show that men work 40 - 60 hrs a week, and women with kids work 168 hrs a week!!!! So now you know why you have jaw/head/migraine pain.

Finances (the psychologists tell us 85% of divorces are over finances), if you're in a partnership, you must both work together on this topic. No one person should be in charge.

This is a nice segue into the "Barefoot Investors" book. He talks about trying to move your job into something you love, or have 2 jobs, one that pays the bills and one that you love. He helps describe scripts for asking for a pay rise from your boss. He shows you how to save up for a safety net (mojo = 3 months' worth of bills, that sit in a high interest account for a rainy day - health-mental burnout / divorce / sickness / fire / etc). Then he moves onto how to save for a house, how to pay it off, how to get the cheapest insurances (I saved $1000 when I did this) and how to set up your super (and what the minimum amount is that you need. This really sets my mind at ease).

Finances is a huge part of people's stress and lives. Get it all sorted. This book has about $15000 worth of advice on stuff that should be taught at school. It is written in basic language, and is really funny, as the guy lives on a farm and writes it around his farm life. So, it's not boring accounting stuff. Most important to me, he shows you how to pay off

your mortgage in 6 years!!! Again, its discipline.
National Debt Helpline on 1800 007 007

Toxic family members

When you have no boundaries, you have to start pulling away and spend less time with the people who make you feel sad, until you learn how to have good boundaries.

To start with it is usually very difficult to explain to them why you are not seeing them, but that's ok, you're an adult, you don't need to justify your reason. When they ask, 'oh we don't see you very much anymore', you can just say 'yeah I'm busy with life'.

It is the same as positive parenting. If your family are nice and recognise your boundaries (which means not meddling in your life, when they are not invited to) then organise to catch up with them at a time that feels right.

If they meddle in your life without permission, put you down, are constantly negative, manipulative, addicted to substances etc, then do not see them. Do not answer their calls, do not answer your door.

If they are old, organise support services, you ARE NOT A DOOR MAT. You deserve love and respect, even if you don't know how to verbalise it!!! Xxx

Unfortunately it is usually left up to one sibling to look after parents. Even if you can't get your siblings to help with your parents, you still deserve to be loved and spoken to as an adult.

Most shires have fantastic websites with support services, and great reception teams with links to government services you can apply for if it is too much for you.

When adults behave badly and have temper tantrums at you, you imagine them at 3yrs. And you certainly would not justify your decision to a 3-year-old.

Counsellors and psychologists are excellent at explaining this concept and how to walk through it. Remember boundaries keep you safe and healthy. They do not push people away. They help to keep the sick/unhealthy people away and allow you to attract new people who see the love and light in your personality.

If you can't work out whether someone is safe to be around. A therapist told me, to imagine a 6-year-old in front of that person (i.e. mother, boss etc), if it's not safe for a 6-year-old to be spoken to in that manner, then it is not safe for you. I know it sounds crazy to have to do this exercise, but co dependence and weird parental up bringing due to that parent trauma, can create an inability to discern what is acceptable in your life, even though you can discern it for others.

Simply, co dependence is where the parent brings up a child like a battery, to help them feel better about themselves, as the parent often feels anxious and unsafe and unsure of what to do. A good book to get a feel for this is called "Co - dependence no more, by Melody Beattie."

Do you have a belief in something greater than you or mankind? And did you know it wants good things for you!!! You may call it the universe, Gaia, the planet, energy, atoms in space, God, buddha, angels etc.

This again, is often not spoken about in families, and it is important for the developing brain to know, that you can't work it all out, and you don't have to a solution to everything.

Find something you believe in - quantum physics, faith, religion. But know they all teach a beautiful universal truth. There is something out there greater than you, and it wants great things for you, and most importantly it loves you unconditionally, even if you forget or don't believe it's there!

The science on this is on the website Blue Zones. It is a large study of places where people live the longest in good health. The biggest contributing factor is faith of some sort.

These basic principles teach that there is a greater presence that loves you so much. This is where you fill yourself up with self-love, from the universe, at an infinite amount. No person, place, or thing will EVER fill you up. I wish someone had told me this earlier than 38 years of age!

Once you get this, you never feel lonely or sad, or lost or not fitting in.

Then you must learn to take total responsibility for everything on the planet, all the good, and all the bad. Everything is a reflection of you.

As you are the universe, and your thoughts create the world/reality you live in. This is very important for people to realise we are responsible for everything in our lives. This allows you to open up to the idea of interconnectedness of everyone and everything on the planet. If you hurt something on the planet, it is like cutting your own arm. It helps you slow down and be less reactive in your day to day lives. Like honking your horn when someone doesn't move off from the lights quick enough. Maybe they are in pain, maybe a family member died, we just don't know everything (universal ignorance of all sides of the story in life. Your point, their point, the universes point, you should try and see 12 different points of view!)

It's then important to study the darker sides of our personality, called the shadow self, or "parts work" and learn about the 'saboteur' part of us, the 'victim' part, and how to make friends with them, ask them what they need when they show up in life and embrace them for the information they are trying to bring, usually about safety and how that information can be used to be victorious and allow that social interaction to be a 'win-win' for you and the other person.

You can only do that if you slow your life down, journal, reflect, meditate.

Enjoy your brain evolution, it is a day by day, life journey, not a 6-week course xxx

LEIGH RAY - THE JAW PHYSIO

This information is based on my life's work since 2001 as a physiotherapist, and prior to that half a degree in Human Movement (now known as Exercise Physiology degree), professional development courses & communication from other specialists I regularly use. This cost me thousands of dollars and a lot of courage to sit on specialists' doors and beg for mentorship, which was often not given easily! It took me 8 years of treating just this area for a lot of specialists to start talking to me. I give this information and trust, you will hold my information in a positive light with thanks.

I am also an 'ex' chronic pain suffer myself. In 2017 I 'cured' myself or stopped having symptoms from 4 chronic conditions that medicine couldn't fix (Endometriosis, IBS, chronic fatigue, fibromyalgia). With over 30 years of 7/10 pain daily, waking 20 times a night and many other horrible symptoms too terrible to discuss. I needed someone to tell me all about my whole health, and how my brain interpreted all aspects of life.

To be honest, surgeries and medication made me much worse. After 30 years, I came off all of them, and decided to see what all this brain work was about. Despite being trained in the 'bio-psycho-social model = medicine!! I was not very aware of the psycho-social side.

My biggest turn around, was when 90% of my burning spinal cord pain (which I had all night and all day) stopped when I took my house keys off my mother (she was walking into my house whenever she wanted). Learning about boundaries and co dependence with loving kindness towards me, through psychotherapy, Buddhist philosophy, (as well as diet, correct hormones) was life changing.

It was not easy, and it took 4 years to see changes, as I had a lot to learn, and 'unpack' as they say in counselling.

Prior to all of that, my beautiful family had paid thousands of dollars in physio, massage, podiatry, Pilates, gynaecologists, gut specialists/gastroenterologists, surgeries, medication, and nothing worked.

My gift to you, is all the years of searching, in one simple book. To give you, what I wanted and needed to hear 30 years ago. My hope is that it only takes you 1 - 2 years to shift your mindset for more ease and grace in your life.

RESOURCES & REFERENCES

TMD
https://tmj.org/hope-in-research/landmark-studies/oppera-study/

Migraines
www.ichd-3.org

Watson DH, Drummond PD. Head Pain Referral During Examination of the Neck in Migraine and Tension-Type Headache. Headache 2012;52:1226-1235 (abstract).

Watson DH, Drummond PD. Cervical Referral of Head Pain in Migraineurs: Effects on the Nociceptive Blink Reflex. Headache 2014;54:1035-1045 (full).

Headaches
https://www.ihs-headache.org/

https://www.ihs-headache.org/ichd-guidelines

Watson DH, Drummond PD. Head Pain Referral During Examination of the Neck in Migraine and Tension-Type Headache. Headache 2012;52:1226-1235 (abstract).

Watson DH, Drummond PD. Cervical Referral of Head Pain in Migraineurs: Effects on the Nociceptive Blink Reflex. Headache 2014;54:1035-1045 (full).

(Pain specialists are finding links between some anti-depressant medication and early onset Alzheimer's, make sure you are informed of your medication).

Evidence suggests that exercise and psychological counselling is just as effective as anti-depressants.

https://link.springer.com/article/10.1007/s10880-008-9105-z
or
https://www.researchgate.net/profile/Daniel_Landers/publication/266406071_The_Influence_of_Exercise_on_Mental_Health/links/551431c30cf23203199cfb4f.pdf

Airways, Sleep Studies

Wake-Up Headache Is Associated With Sleep Bruxism - Vieira - 2020 - Headache: The Journal of Head and Face Pain - Wiley Online Library.

Tarja Saaresranta 1, Olli Polo. Hormones and Breathing, Chest. 2002 Dec;122(6):2165-82. doi: 10.1378/chest.122.6.2165.

Diet, Gut Health

www.anhinternational.org

'Research confirms gut-brain connection in autism' - news release May 2019/EurekAlert (credit RMIT University).

Dr William Davis website (Cardiologist, Author, and Health Crusader). 'Essential oils for fungal overgrowth', by Dr Davis, Jan 17th 2019.

Green Med Info. The Science of Natural Healing. 'Research proves wheat can cause harm to everyone's intestines. Oct 2nd 2013.

www.gutfoundation.com.au

neurosciencenews.com, 'Gut bacteria linked to Depression Identified' Feb 4th 2019. Summary: A new study reports two different gut bacteria are depleted in people with depression, regardless of antidepressant treatments.

Dr William Davis website (Cardiologist, Author, and Health Crusader). 'Essential oils for fungal overgrowth', by Dr Davis, Jan 17th 2019.

Green Med Info. The Science of Natural Healing. 'Research proves wheat can cause harm to everyone's intestines. Oct 2nd 2013.

Hormones

Period repair manual (Book), by Lara Briden.

https://www.amazon.com/gp/product/0984187731/ref=dbs_a_def_rwt_bibl_vppi_i1

Books from Dr Dan Purser (Endometriosis, Healthy menopause, Vitamin deficiencies, Resolving Osteoporosis, Breast Cancer Survival Guide, Thyroid Problems, Fibromyalgia, Progesterone, Improving Men's sexuality and testosterone, and more.

https://www.amazon.com/Dan-Purser-MD/e/B00BIKSGVQ/ref=sr_ntt_srch_lnk_1?qid=1517000404&sr=8-1

Endometriosis and PMS
Facebook video from Dr Dan Purser; *https://www.facebook.com/watch/live/?v=326757721338428&ref=watch_permalink*

https://danpursermd.com/

Lab Ranges
Purser+Lab+Solutions+v2.pdf

General Health and all conditions
A Patients guide on proactive preventative Medicine, Program 120, Female handbook

A Patients guide on proactive preventative Medicine, Program 120, Male handbook, by Dr Dan Purser.

https://danpursermd.com/

https://danpursermd.com/downloads

Cowan LD, Gordis L, et al. Breast cancer incidence in women with a history of progesterone deficiency. Am J Epidemiol. 1981.

Brain Evolution,Mmindfulness
The secret language of your body, by Inna Segal.

The body keeps the score, by Bessel van der Kolk.

Co dependence no more, by Melodie Beattie.

The Inner Child Workbook, by Cathryn L Taylor.

Homecoming, by John Bradshaw.

https://www.freedomfromchronicpain.com/

www.ingramcontent.com/pod-product-compliance
Lightning Source LLC
Chambersburg PA
CBHW072154020426
42334CB00018B/1996